RETURNING MATERIALS:
Place in book drop to
remove this checkout from
your record. FINES will
be charged if book is
returned after the date

Agricultural Uses of Antibiotics

ACS SYMPOSIUM SERIES **320**

Agricultural Uses of Antibiotics

William A. Moats, EDITOR
U.S. Department of Agriculture

Developed from a symposium sponsored by
the Division of Agricultural and Food Chemistry
at the 190th Meeting
of the American Chemical Society,
Chicago, Illinois,
September 8–13, 1985

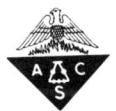

American Chemical Society, Washington, DC 1986

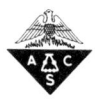

Library of Congress Cataloging-in-Publication Data
Agricultural uses of antibiotics.
(ACS symposium series, ISSN 0097-6156; 320)

"Developed from a symposium sponsored by the Division of Agriculture and Food Chemistry at the 190th Meeting of the American Chemical Society, Chicago, Illinois, September 8-13, 1985."

Includes bibliographies and indexes.

1. Antibiotics in veterinary medicine—Congresses.
2. Antibiotics in agriculture—Congresses. 3. Antibiotics in animal nutrition—Congresses. 4. Antibiotic residues—Hygienic aspects—Congresses. 5. Food contamination—Congresses.

I. Moats, William A. (William Alden),1928-
II. American Chemical Society. Division of Agricultural and Food Chemistry. III. American Chemical Society. Meeting (190th: 1985: Chicago, Ill.)
IV. Series. [DNLM: 1. Agriculture—congresses.
2. Antibiotics—congresses. 3. Food Contamination—congresses. 4. Veterinary Medicine—congresses.
QV 350 A278 1985]

SF918.A5A37   1986   663.1'929   86-20614
ISBN 0-8412-0996-0

Copyright © 1986
American Chemical Society

All Rights Reserved. The appearance of the code at the bottom of the first page of each chapter in this volume indicates the copyright owner's consent that reprographic copies of the chapter may be made for personal or internal use or for the personal or internal use of specific clients. This consent is given on the condition, however, that the copier pay the stated per copy fee through the Copyright Clearance Center, Inc., 27 Congress Street, Salem, MA 01970, for copying beyond that permitted by Sections 107 or 108 of the U.S. Copyright Law. This consent does not extend to copying or transmission by any means—graphic or electronic—for any other purpose, such as for general distribution, for advertising or promotional purposes, for creating a new collective work, for resale, or for information storage and retrieval systems. The copying fee for each chapter is indicated in the code at the bottom of the first page of the chapter.

The citation of trade names and/or names of manufacturers in this publication is not to be construed as an endorsement or as approval by ACS of the commercial products or services referenced herein; nor should the mere reference herein to any drawing, specification, chemical process, or other data be regarded as a license or as a conveyance of any right or permission, to the holder, reader, or any other person or corporation, to manufacture, reproduce, use, or sell any patented invention or copyrighted work that may in any way be related thereto. Registered names, trademarks, etc., used in this publication, even without specific indication thereof, are not to be considered unprotected by law.

PRINTED IN THE UNITED STATES OF AMERICA

ACS Symposium Series

M. Joan Comstock, *Series Editor*

Advisory Board

Harvey W. Blanch
University of California—Berkeley

Alan Elzerman
Clemson University

John W. Finley
Nabisco Brands, Inc.

Marye Anne Fox
The University of Texas—Austin

Martin L. Gorbaty
Exxon Research and Engineering Co.

Roland F. Hirsch
U.S. Department of Energy

Rudolph J. Marcus
Consultant, Computers &
 Chemistry Research

Vincent D. McGinniss
Battelle Columbus Laboratories

Donald E. Moreland
USDA, Agricultural Research Service

W. H. Norton
J. T. Baker Chemical Company

James C. Randall
Exxon Chemical Company

W. D. Shults
Oak Ridge National Laboratory

Geoffrey K. Smith
Rohm & Haas Co.

Charles S. Tuesday
General Motors Research Laboratory

Douglas B. Walters
National Institute of
 Environmental Health

C. Grant Willson
IBM Research Department

FOREWORD

The ACS SYMPOSIUM SERIES was founded in 1974 to provide a medium for publishing symposia quickly in book form. The format of the Series parallels that of the continuing ADVANCES IN CHEMISTRY SERIES except that, in order to save time, the papers are not typeset but are reproduced as they are submitted by the authors in camera-ready form. Papers are reviewed under the supervision of the Editors with the assistance of the Series Advisory Board and are selected to maintain the integrity of the symposia; however, verbatim reproductions of previously published papers are not accepted. Both reviews and reports of research are acceptable, because symposia may embrace both types of presentation.

CONTENTS

Preface ix

1. Antibiotics Use in Agriculture: An Overview 1
   Richard H. Gustafson

USES

2. Therapeutic Use of Antibiotics in Farm Animals 8
   G. Ziv

3. Antibiotics in Treatment of Mastitis 23
   W. D. Schultze

4. Antibiotics in Beekeeping 35
   Robert J. Argauer

5. Antibiotics as Crop Protectants 49
   Arun K. Misra

6. Trends in the Use of Fermentation Products in Agriculture 61
   R. W. Burg

RISKS AND BENEFITS

7. Benefits and Risks of Antibiotics Use in Agriculture 74
   Virgil W. Hays

8. Significance of Antibiotics in Foods and Feeds 88
   Khem M. Shahani and Paul J. Whalen

9. Risks to Human Health from the Use of Antibiotics in Animal Feeds ... 100
   Philip J. Frappaolo

10. Effects of Low Levels of Antibiotics in Livestock Feeds 112
    Thomas H. Jukes

RESIDUES

11. Antibiotic Residues in Food: Regulatory Aspects 128
    Robert C. Livingston

12. The U.S. Department of Agriculture Meat and Poultry Antibiotic Residue Testing Program 137
    Bernard Schwab and Jeffrey Brown

13. Microbiological Assay Procedures for Antibiotic Residues 142
    Stanley E. Katz

14. Physicochemical Methods for Identifying Antibiotic Residues in Foods 154
    William A. Moats

15. Pharmacokinetics and Residues of Sulfadimidine and Its N^4-Acetyl and Hydroxy Metabolites in Food-Producing Animals 168
    J. F. M. Nouws, T. B. Vree, R. Aerts, and J. Grondel

INDEXES

Author Index 184

Subject Index 184

PREFACE

ANTIBIOTICS ORDINARILY ARE DEFINED as antibacterial or antiparasitic compounds derived from microorganisms. In this book sulfonamides also are included because, while they are not derived from microorganisms, they are used in the same manner as antibiotics.

Since the discovery of penicillin, an enormous number of antibiotic compounds have been isolated. They have found uses both in treatment of human disease and in various aspects of agriculture, including treatment of animal and plant diseases, and as feed additives to promote growth of animals. Some antibiotics such as tylosin were developed specifically for agricultural use.

This book was developed to provide a current perspective on agricultural use of antibiotics. Topics include some major uses of antibiotics, problems associated with their use from a regulatory standpoint, residues in food including methods of detection, risks to human health from use in feeds, trends in use, and overall risks and benefits. The scope, therefore, is much broader than in several other recent symposia that have focused mainly on the controversy regarding the use of antibiotics as feed additives. Many of the topics included in the present volume have not been discussed under one cover before.

The practice of incorporating low levels of antibiotics in livestock feeds to promote growth has been particularly controversial. It is feared that this practice will result in development of resistant bacteria in animals, which will in turn be passed on to humans, thus diminishing the effectiveness of antibiotics in treatment of human disease. A petition from the Natural Resources Defense Council to ban such uses of penicillin and tetracyclines recently was denied by the Secretary of Health and Human Services. The controversy therefore is likely to continue. Opinion on the subject is quite polarized, and several points of view are presented in this book.

Thanks are due to participants in the symposium for their support and diligence in preparing the material for publication and to the ACS Books Department for their unfailing support and guidance.

WILLIAM A. MOATS
Meat Science Research Laboratory
Agricultural Research Service
U.S. Department of Agriculture
Beltsville, MD 20705

Antibiotics Use in Agriculture: An Overview

Richard H. Gustafson

Agricultural Research Division, American Cyanamid Company, Princeton, NJ 08540

Antimicrobial agents and antibiotics in particular have been utilized in livestock rearing for more than thirty years. This has allowed the production of meat, eggs, and milk at levels of efficiency significantly higher than that seen in the pre-antibiotic era. In terms of current kilogram amounts in the U.S., the feed additive uses far surpass all other uses in agriculture and approach the total amount utilized in human medicine. Starting in the 1960's, the use of antibiotic feed additives has been questioned by some as a potential threat to human health. This long standing controversy has been a difficult one for regulatory officials, scientific advisory groups, and legislators who must decide whether directed changes in current agricultural uses are justified.

The use of antibiotics in agriculture is a subject of wide variety and complexities. It is also a subject of considerable controversy. It was in the years surrounding 1950 that Dr. Jukes and his colleagues demonstrated that chlortetracycline at low levels, i.e. 20 ppm and lower, could improve performance in livestock (1). By performance we mean the rate of gain and the amount of feed per unit of gain. Antibiotics, particularly penicillin, had been used in animals prior to that period, but only as an injectable in sick livestock or as mammary infusions in lactating dairy animals suffering from mastitis. After Stokstad and Jukes opened the door and many agricultural researchers walked in, the development of antimicrobials as feed additives developed at a rapid pace (2).

Registration and Commercialization

Today, in the United States, the FDA is responsible for examining safety and efficacy data before an antibiotic or synthetic chemical may be commercialized for livestock use. This includes studies on formulations, product stability, conventional and genetic toxicity, environmental safety, metabolism, residue studies in target animals, studies on antibiotic resistance in gut microflora and on salmonella shedding in target animals. Similar requirements are part of registering these products in overseas markets. In general, after a product is discovered in the laboratory, many years and millions of dollars are required to bring it to commercialization. Extending registrations of existing products to other livestock species is also a time-consuming and expensive proposition. The big three meat species are poultry, swine, and cattle. The potential markets for these groups of animals may support the required industrial research if the probability of registration and commercial success are high. On the other hand, the minor species, goats, sheep, turkeys, cultured fish often do not support large expensive programs. The dairy industry is also large and antibiotics for the control of mastitis must be considered a significant market. Antibiotics to be used as feed additives must also be inexpensive and fermentation yields often need to be improved before commercialization is possible. Some feed additives are used as biomass products. They are marketed this way because the high costs of extensive purification would make any other course impractical. A biomass product contains the inert spent products of fermentation, remnants of the producing organism, media, precipitation products, etc.

The following demonstrates the number of registered feed additives according to category.

Table I. The Number of Registered Feed Additives According to Category

Synthetic		Antibiotic	
13	Anticoccidials	3	Anticoccidials
5	Antibacterials	14	Antibacterials
4	Histomonastats	1	Anthelmintic
8	Anthelmintics		
9	Miscellaneous		

Antibiotic is defined here as a chemical produced in whole or in part by a microorganism in large scale fermentation. Definitions after that are somewhat grey. For example, two of the three ionophore anticoccidials currently used by the poultry industry are also used to promote feed efficiency in cattle, and that effect is certainly a consequence of antibacterial activity in the rumen. Many of the narrow spectrum gram positive antibiotics are poorly absorbed from the gut and registration claims are confined to growth promotion and feed efficiency, particularly at the commonly used levels. Other antibiotics are well absorbed and provide a significant measure of protection against bacterial disease, in addition to promoting growth and feed efficiency. It should be noted that although the summary table provides information on the variety of products which are available, the list doesn't necessarily reflect current uses. For example, synthetic chemicals dominated the anticoccidial market during the 1950's and 60's. With the introduction of monensin, the first ionophore antibiotic used for this purpose the anticoccidial market shifted away from synthetic chemicals and toward antibiotics, where it exists today. Nevertheless, the older synthetic products are still registered and are still part of the armamentarium of anticoccidials. There are more than twice as many synthetic chemicals as antibiotics registered for feed additive use. Table II lists antibacterial drugs, fermentation products and synthesized chemicals approved for use in food animals.

Table II. Antibacterial Feed Additives

Synthetic	Antibiotic
Carbodox	Bacitracin Methylene Disalicylate
Furazolidone	Bacitracin Zinc
Nitrofurazone	Bambermycins
Sulfamethazine	Chlortetracycline
Sulfathiazole	Erythromycin
	Lincomycin
	Neomycin
	Novobiocin
	Nystatin
	Oxytetracycline
	Penicillin
	Streptomycin
	Tylosin
	Virginiamycin

The nitrofurans and sulfa drugs are antibacterial feed additives that occupy a continuing important position in the prophylaxis and treatment of livestock disease. These are products which are well absorbed and have good activity against a variety of respiratory pathogens. Carbadox, another synthetic feed additive, has been used extensively in the swine industry for performance improvement and the control of swine dysentery.

Uses of Antibiotics in Animal Agriculture

The antibiotic feed additives era started with the tetracyclines and this class continues to dominate the field. Chlortetracycline and oxytetracycline were initially used at fairly low levels as promoters of growth and feed efficiency. As the market for these products increased rapidly, production efficicency and fermentation yields also improved. Eventually costs came down and it was economically feasible to use them at higher levels in poultry, swine and cattle, i.e. prophylactic levels which controlled endemic bacterial diseases. A combination for swine was introduced in the 1960's, consisting of chlortetracycline at 100 g/ton, sulfamethazine at 100 g/ton, and penicillin G at 50 g/ton and it was the rapid acceptance of this product by swine producers which was partially responsible for an upsurge of antibiotic use in livestock production. At the same time tetracyclines became increasingly useful in protecting feedlot cattle from the bacterial component of respiratory diseases, as well as reducing the prevalence of liver abscesses caused by Fusobacterium. Anaplasmosis is controlled by tetracyclines in those areas where this disease is endemic in cattle. The poultry industry has also used tetracyclines at higher levels to protect flocks against respiratory diseases as well as controlling certain enteric infections. These prophylactic uses are used particularly at times and in animals in which the risk of bacterial disease is highest. This high risk situation tends to operate in young animals, or when livestock, particularly cattle, are exposed to the stresses of shipment or severe weather. It should be noted that injectable antibiotics are also used extensively in feedlot cattle with a penicillin-streptomycin combination and injectable oxytetracycline used rather extensively for respiratory disease.

The current uses of tetracyclines in the poultry industry are almost entirely at the higher levels for the control of bacterial disease. This includes both feed additive and drinking water formulations.

Tylosin and erythromycin are commonly used in the livestock industry. These macrolides show wide spectrum activity against gram positive organisms with particularly useful activity against mycoplasma in poultry, swine, and cattle. The combination of tylosin and sulfamethazine is used in swine feed. Erythromycin, the first commercialized macrolide and long the flagship of this group in human medicine, is also registered for use in poultry, swine, and cattle but is used far less than tylosin. Both erythromycin and tylosin are also used therapeutically as injectables and in drinking water for treatment of a variety of infections.

The only beta-lactam antibiotics used in food producing animals are penicillin G, ampicillin, amoxicillin, hetacillin, cloxacillin, and cephapiron. Of these, only penicillin G is used as a feed additive, most of it as a combination product in the swine industry. Penicillin feed additives are also registered for use in poultry, but not in cattle. Although penicillin has negligible activity against most gram negative organisms, later generations of beta-lactams have had a much broader spectrum. This group of antibiotics has been the subject of a great deal of pharmaceutical company research, primarily because of the existence in nature of a wide variety of beta-lactamases and cephalosporinases, enzymes which break down various members of this class. Beta-lactam antibiotics continue to be in the forefront of human medicine and as mammary infusion products in the dairy industry.

Aminoglycosides registered for feed additive use include streptomycin and neomycin although these antibiotics currently are not being used extensively. Gentamicin and kanamycin are not registered for feed use but are approved as injectables. Gentamicin is also used in an egg dip solution to control specific pathogens in the turkey industry.

The general group of antibiotics characterized by gram positive activity and poor absorption from the gut are used principally for growth promotion and feed efficiency in the swine and poultry industry. These include bacitracin, the bambermycins, and virginiamycin. In addition, two products of this type used freqently in Europe and the Far East are avoparcin and nitrovin. The growth promoters major claims are for improved rate of gain and feed efficiency, although occcasionally claims at high levels for disease control have been allowed. For example, virginiamycin is registered at 25 to 100 grams/ton for control of swine dysentery in the United States. In the European Economic Community, these growth promoters are used free sale, strictly for performance purposes and disease claims are not made. Therapeutic and prophylactic feed additives for the control of bacterial infections are used by veterinary order.

Although the feed additive uses of antibiotics have been emphasized, it should be noted that the uses as injectables for therapy, mammary infusions for mastitis, boluses, pills, capsules, medicated blocks, and drinking water formulations include a wider variety of antibiotics than are added to feeds. Many of these are currently used at the discretion of the meat producer or dairyman, others must be used under the direction of a veterinarian. For example, chloramphenicol is an antibiotic which the veterinarian has access to, but which the FDA has indicated should not be used in livestock destined for human consumption, primarily because of the

Agency's concern about the potential for toxic residues in humans. This antibiotic is used in European livestock.

Extent of Antibiotic Use

A question which should be considered here is the extent of antibiotic use in meat production. It's difficult to obtain market figures on individual antibiotic products since the industry considers this information proprietary. It is also unclear how to best express the extent of agricultural uses. Should we be talking about dollars or kilograms? There is no doubt that in terms of kilograms, feed additive use is by far the most significant. The National Academy of Sciences in their 1980 report on feed antibiotics (3) cited figures obtained from the U.S. International Trade Commission, showing non-medical uses to be between 5 and 6 million kilograms in 1978. Unfortunately reporting by weight tends to blur the distinction between growth promoters which are used at 3 or 4 grams per ton such as the bambermycins, and coccidiostats such as monensin, which are used at 100 g/ton. The differences in feed consumption by chickens, swine, and cattle also compound the difficulty of examining antibiotic use. According to figures released by the Animal Health Institute, 1983 sales by American companies of pharmaceuticals, biologicals, and feed additives for animal agriculture exceeded 2 billion dollars (4). These figures represent sales at the manufacturers level. The total feed additive market for 1983 was about half of that total. Pharmaceutical antibacterials sold for $210 million and animal feed antibacterials at $271 million that year. In terms of value to the consumer, the Council of Agricultural Science and Technology reviewed six economic studies and concluded that feed additives save the U.S. consumer approximately $3.5 billion per year in meat prices (5). Antibiotic use accounts for most of this. Although specific figures are proprietary, the tetracyclines have dominated the product lists in terms of total use but tylosin, sulfa drugs, nitrofurans, the gram positive growth promoters and the ionophore antibiotics are also highly significant.

The Public Health Question

The long controversy surrounding antibiotic feed additives is principally concerned with selection of antibiotic resistant bacteria in livestock. The public health significance under consideration may be reduced to the following questions: "Do the uses of antibiotics in meat animals interfere with the continued efficacy of antibiotics in human medicine?" and secondly, if there is a connection, "would stricter controls on certain feed additive uses help maintain antibiotic effectiveness?" In the United States, the controversy has currently settled on feed additive uses of tetracyclines and penicillin. In response to similar concerns in England in the 1960's, the Swann Committee recommended that feed additives used only for growth promotion and feed efficiency continue to be permitted free sale but that antibiotics used for prevention or control of disease be used only on veterinary prescription. These regulations were implemented in England in 1971 and a few years later, by several other European countries. Most observers agree that these regulations have not altered antibiotic resistance levels in livestock and that antibiotics having disease claims continue to be widely used in these countries, even though veterinary prescriptions are required. The veal calf industry overseas uses antibiotics in milk replacer in order to protect the health of these young animals which are particularly susceptible to stress and bacterial infections.

The FDA and industry have both been embroiled in the antibiotic resistance controversy for more than 15 years and a resolution of the dispute remains elusive. Part of the reason is that the subject is highly politicized with pressures on the FDA from a variety of sources anxious to introduce new restrictions. The communications media, TV, newspapers, periodicals have also turned their attention to this subject in recent years. Agricultural groups, industry manufacturers, and congressmen with agricultural constituencies have tended to remind the FDA that restrictions are not justified so pressure on the Agency comes from both sides of the issue. It's my opinion that most microbiologists, infectious disease experts, and epidemiologists believe that further government restrictions on the agricultural use of antibiotics would accomplish nothing in the way of public health benefits.

This overview has presented an introduction to the subject of antibiotics in animal agriculture and provides a general view of the extent of antibiotic use. The manuscripts to follow will offer more details and provide additional food for thought. Certainly the current efficient production of meat and dairy products is dependent on a wide variety of antibiotics and this will continue to be true in most Western countries in which livestock production is an important part of the economy.

Literature Cited

1. Stokstad, E. L. R.; Jukes, T. H., Proc. Soc. Exptl. Biol. Med., 73; 523-528.
2. Gustafson, R. H.; Kiser, J. S., In "The Tetracycline"; Hlavka, J. J.; Boothe, J. H., Eds; HANDBOOK EXP. PHARM.; Springer-Verlag: Heidelberg, 1985; pp. 405-446.
3. "The Effects on Human Health of Subtherapeutic Use of Antimicrobials in Animal Feeds". National Academy of Sciences, National Research Council; Washington, March 1980.
4. Animal Health Institute; 119 Oronoco St., Alexandria, VA.
5. "Antibiotics in Animal Feeds"; Council for Agricultural Science and Technology, Report No. 88, March 1981.

RECEIVED February 19, 1986

USES

# 2

Therapeutic Use of Antibiotics in Farm Animals

G. Ziv

Ministry of Agriculture, Kimron Veterinary Institute, P.O. Box 12, Bet Dagan, Israel

The prevention and therapeutic management of disease conditions caused by infectious agents are daily events in the practice of farm animal medicine and surgery. Antimicrobial drugs represent one third of all chemicals used in veterinary medicine. The use of antimicrobials by practitioners involves therapy of bovine species, 75%, compared with 25% for the treatment of infections in horses, pigs and other farm animals. Antimicrobials are used to treat mastitis, enteritis, peritonitis, metritis, pneumonia, septicemia, and localized infections. The successful use of these agents for each indication depends on the same basic principles that apply to all microbial infections: (i) identifying the incriminating pathogen, (ii) determining the in vitro sensitivity of the pathogen to the antibacterial drug, (iii) attaining and maintaining therapeutic drug concentrations at the infection site, (iv) minimizing local and systemic side-effects of therapy, and (v) the administration of supportive, non-antimicrobial, therapy when indicated. Pharmacokinetic and pharmaceutical properties, cost, and duration of drug residues are also important criteria for drug selection. Antimicrobial therapy is generally applied on a herd basis in order that animals returned to full health and productivity at the earliest opportunity, that the excretion of pathogenic organisms from sick animals be curtailed, and that epidemics of infectious diseases be prevented from developing.

Antibiotics are used for many purposes in agriculture but perhaps the most important of these uses is that for the maintenance of health in our food animal population. Essentially, antimicrobial agents are used to treat disease, to prevent the spread of infection, and to check the multiplication of tissue-associated infective agents. Antibiotics are very complex therapeutic tools and their correct use requires a wide knowledge of physiology, pathology, pharmacology, diagnostics and legislation. A proper acquaintance

0097-6156/86/0320-0008$06.00/0
© 1986 American Chemical Society

with these disciplines enables the veterinary practitioner to apply antibiotics in a manner that will ensure their continued safe and effective use for the treatment and prevention of diseases in farm animals.

The treatment of bacterial diseases in man and companion animals is invariably directed at the individual patient whereas in food producing animals, especially pigs and sheep, although a degree of individual therapy may be undertaken, antimicrobial therapy is generally applied on a herd or flock basis. Present-day antimicrobial substances are very sophisticated tools in the armory of the veterinary practitioner and animal producer. Use of these substances in the field may appear to the novice very simple and free from any attendant hazard, yet this is only true when these drugs are being used by persons fully conversant with their pharmacological properties and thus able to avoid such problems as tissue residues and certain direct toxic affects.

Rationale for use of antibiotics

Any individual, group or population of animals is always susceptible to outbreaks of clinical disease. Many present-day agricultural practices such as livestock marketing, movement of very young animals and certain forms of intensification can act as trigger factors for the initiation and development of clinical diseases (1). Generally speaking, disease will be more prevalent in large groups of intensively managed animals than in individual animals kept under extensive conditions. Over the years new animal hybrids have been developed, highly productive strains of livestock have been bred, and imported breeds have been introduced into new localities with the sole intention of increasing productivity and quality of animal products. This has resulted in some cases in an increase prevalence of disease which has to be constantly treated or prevented. In order to cut down economic losses it is necessary that bacterial disease be treated as soon as possible with an antibacterial agent. Present-day economics dictates that animals be returned to full health and productivity at the earliest opportunity, that the excretion and dissemination of pathogenic organisms from sick animals be curtailed, and that epidemics of infectious diseases be prevented from developing (2). Any delay in the administration of antibacterials, either to the individual or to a herd, will be counter-productive and economically unsound. Antibacterial drugs were developed with the sole purpose of helping to treat sick farm animals afflicted with bacterial disease and in so doing the dissemination of pathogenic micro-organisms within the common environment of man and animals would be very much reduced and in some cases totally prevented.

It would not be difficult to speculate on the problems that would arise if no antibacterial medication were available. Large numbers of farm animals would perish, chronic bacterial disease would be commonplace and the consequent losses both of life and productivity would drastically inflate the cost of milk and meat production apart from resulting in the bankruptcy and disappearance of many livestock producers.

Epidemiological experience has shown that the introduction of an infectious disease-causing agent into a large group of susceptible animals in the same pen will ultimately result in a large proportion of these animals becoming infected (3, 4). The rational therapeutic approach to this problem is to treat the whole group as an individual. In this way one avoids having to continually withdraw and treat individual animals which would be very costly in time and also stressful to the animals due to frequent interference by the human attendants when catching animals for medication. The concept of herd medication is difficult to accept outside the agricultural field. The experience of veterinary practitioners who treat large herds of animals, however, fully supports the practice of herd medication, especially in those areas of animal management where it is essential to keep all the animals at a level of optimal productivity (2). Extensive experience in veterinary medicine has clearly indicated the need for such treatment, especially when highly infectious or contagious diseases are involved. It must be realized that unlike the human family unit, all the farm animals in a group that is being managed under intensive systems are usually of the same age, usually very immature, and are in constant contact with their faeces.

Another factor which presently produces continuing disease problems in calf and pig enterprises is the need to transfer young growing animals from breeding units to the grower/finisher units. This frequently involves prolonged travelling, a change in diet and a mixing together of animals from different sources. Inevitably this can culminate in a disturbance of the gastro-intestinal flora which is caused by dietary change, reorganisation of social dominance (pecking order), and redistribution of micro-organisms of many species and types within the newly grouped animals. Such disturbances frequently result in the production of overt clinical disease. A similar set of circumstances also may occur at weaning. These events are usually totally predictable and experience has shown that, under certain circumstances, if pre-emptive medication is not applied then serious health problems will ensue.

The decision to employ herd medication is never taken lightly because of the cost of the drugs to treat a large population of animals and the problems which will ensue with the need to adhere to drug withdrawal times. Herd medication on a very large scale also involves such logistical problems as getting the correct dose of drug to all individuals concerned and the difficulties of being able to obtain a very large amount of drug when required and without delay. Care is also required in the choice and use of antibiotics for the treatment of zoonotic infections, e.g. salmonellosis. Some manifestations of this disease are more amenable to treatment than others and special considerations have to be taken in order to avoid undue selection of multiple antibiotic resistance and destruction of indigenous protective microflora.

A further extention of herd medication has often in the past been referred to as prophylactic treatment or disease prevention. Both terms are partially correct but the rationale for their application requires a basic knowledge of epidemiology. The application of pre-emptive medication depends upon the knowledge that a particular bacterial agent has been introduced into a population and is causing clinical disease in individuals within that population (5). Previous veterinary experience will have indicated that if medication is not applied to the group or herd then there will be a continuing sequence of infected individuals, accompanied by a prolonged period of sub-optimal performance in the affected group of animals. Generally speaking, pre-emptive medication does not apply to the individually housed animal but only to the group or herd of animals in which clinical disease has broken out in one or more individuals. Rapid curtailment of a herd infection will bring about a cessation of bacterial excretion which will be advantageous to the remainder of the herd and also prevent undue contamination of the farm environment. An example of pre-emptive medication is the use of dry-cow therapy in which a slow release antibiotic preparation is infused into the cow's udder at the end of a lactation to overcome any residual infection and to protect against the establishment of new infection during the dry period and prior to the commencement of a new lactation cycle (2).

Selection of antibiotics

The selection and use of antibiotics in clinical practice are dependant upon many factors, not the least of which are the particular drug use habits in the geographical area (6). Because the majority of bacterial pathogens are susceptible to several antibiotics, successful therapy should not be unexpected with different drug use patterns. There are, however, some important factors which should be given consideration when selecting antibacterial agents. Bacterial sensitivity is a prominent decision factor which is commonly of high priority. However, of nearly equal importance is the ability of the drug to achieve reasonable concentrations at the site of infection. Additionally, the age and health state of the animal should also be considered along with dosage preparations available, cost, toxicity, etc. Therapy shall fail with the use of a very potent oral antibiotic which does not penetrate into the site of infection or which is degraded by ruminal microflora before it can be absorbed. The lipid solubility and degree of ionization at physiological pH of the drug are important determinants of tissue penetration. Generally, the more lipid-soluble drugs which are little ionized at physiological pH are more widely distributed in the body and are most likely to achieve reasonable concentrations in difficult-to-penetrate peripheral tissues such as brain and reproductive tract. The pH of the tissue is also important since tissues with a pH lower than that of blood (7.4) will trap basic antibiotics in them by causing increased ionization of the antibiotic. An example of this is the mammary gland with a pH of 6.8 to 7.0. In this case the basic macrolide antibiotics which are lipid-soluble and are little ionized in blood will be found in higher levels in milk than some less lipid-soluble drugs because they are trapped in the acidic milk and move from blood into milk more readily than from milk to blood. Conversely, acidic antibiotics may be found in lower than expected concentrations in tissues with a pH lower than blood. As a general rule, these relationships can be used to determine the need for dosage adjustment for infections involving specific tissues. In situations where an antibiotic is known to penetrate specific tissues poorly, the dosage may need to be increased appropriately.

After an antibiotic was selected, the primary concern should be to optimize the dosage for maximal efficacy and minimal toxicity. Other factors such as economics, frequency of animal handling and route of administration are important for both dosage determination and drug selection. Often, because of cost or inadequate animal dosage information, the tendency is to use too low dosages which may be quite sufficient in some cases but in others may lead to the erroneous conclusion that the drug is not effective. The dose may actually be appropriate but the dosage interval too long to sustain activity, or the opposite situation with dose too low and interval appropriate.

A desired serum or tissue concentration can be determined from the in vitro bacterial sensitivity data. It is generally desirable to select a dosage schedule which will provide serum or tissue levels equal to or exceeding in in vitro inhibitory concentrations for a substantial portion of the treatment period. For some bacteria low antibacterial concentrations may suffice if the more sensitive organisms are involved. Yet the next instance of disease encountered due to the same organism may be refractory to all but the highest doses of drug. Once a desired serum or tissue level has been decided, the dosage schedule may be determined. If the dosage schedule fails to provide the appropriate serum level, adjustments can be made accordingly. In some cases an increase in dose will provide a proportional increase in serum concentration. This is true for intravenous preparations and for intramuscular administration of some water-soluble antibiotics such as the aminoglycosides. Shortening the dosage interval may in some cases provide sufficient increase in serum concentration. Unfortunately, the relationship between dosage and serum concentration is not readily predictable in some cases with oral or intramuscular administration. This is particularly true for slow-absorption formulations such as procaine penicillin G, ampicillin trihydrate, and some oxytetracycline injectable products. In these cases increasing the dose will more effectively increase the duration of action rather than serum concentrations. If the situation demands infrequent drug administration, the dose must be increased too. In most cases this does not present a toxicity problem because toxicity is usually due to cumulative effects of the drug, as with the aminoglycosides and polymyxins.

The foregoing comments are based on the ultimate objective of antibacterial therapy, attainment of adequate tissue drug levels to either kill the pathogen or inhibit its growth. Adequate tissue levels are usually interpreted as levels equivalent or higher than the minimal inhibitory concentrations (MIC) of the drug as determined by standardized in vitro procedures. The most readily available tissue for analysis and one which is in equilibrium with most other tissues is serum. Hence, serum levels of antibiotics are often used as an indication of adequacy of dosage. This relationship is not infallible, however, since other factors may also play important roles. The state of body defense mechanisms may significantly alter the efficacy of a given serum or tissue level. Thus the interpretation of in vivo studies with antimicrobial agents is complicated by the importance of the host defenses in producing the final cure. The host defenses probably have a more dominant role in the outcome when bacteriostatic antibiotics like tetracyclines, chloramphenicol and sulfonamides are used than with bactericidally acting antibiotics like the beta-lactam and aminoglycoside antibiotics. This is probably true in most clinical situations. The amount of drug required to kill a certain bacterial strain may vary depending on the number of organisms in the inoculum. This has been termed the inoculum effect, and although its clinical importance is not fully understood, the effect is known to vary with the drug used and the bacterium being treated. Additionally, in some instances serum levels may not accurately reflect tissue levels, especially with antibiotics with high tissue levels, such as the macrolides (6).

With the exception of some highly sensitive bacterial isolates and a few sustained-release formulations of antimicrobial drugs, it is usually necessary to administer multiple doses of a drug to control an infection. However, at the present time, it is not established for most infections whether it is better to achieve high levels of drug in serum rapidly and thereby achieve high levels in tissues, or whether it is more desirable to have a drug present for a long period, albeit at lower levels. There are virtually no well-controlled comparisons of these different situations (7).

Concentrations of antimicrobial agents that are below the MIC but produce morphologic or quantitative alternations in micro-organisms are defined as subinhibitory concentrations. Effects of sub-MIC of antimicrobial agents include: (i) alternation of structure of micro-organisms, (ii) alternation of numbers of micro-organisms, (iii) alternation of adhesiveness to mucosal surfaces, (iv) enhancement of phagocytosis or impairment of expression of antiphagocytic material, and (v) induction of beta-lactamase production by the bacterium (8). Additional studies are needed to define the true clinical importance of the sub-MIC, post-antibiotic effect, post-antibiotic leukocyte enhancement, and greatly fluctuating serum drug concentrations. The preponderance of evidence, although much of it empirical, indicates that tissue and/or blood concentrations that are equal to or above the MIC should be attained, especially with bacteriostatic-type antimicrobial agents or in animals with refractory type of infections. Since the ultimate test of antibiotic effectiveness is the response of the animal, the use of serum levels for predicting efficacy is only as valuable as its ability to predict the response of the whole animal (6). Generally, this correlation has held, hence the use of serum levels for determination of antibiotic usage. The fore-going limitations should, however, be kept in perspective while using such information clinically.

The situation with the sulfonamides is quite different than with many of the antibiotics. In this instance the correlation between attainment of _in vitro_ inhibitory concentration requirements as _in vivo_ serum concentrations and drug efficacy has not been as good as with most of the antibiotics. As a result, a general recommendation of 50 ug/ml of drug in serum has been widely accepted as the desirable concentration for all the sulfonamides. Unfortunately little effort has been expended in veterinary medicine to determine MIC relationships between various bacteria and sulfonamides (6).

An important principle to be emphasized is that there is no single optimal dose for any given antibiotic. There are too many variables such as host resistance, bacterial virulence, bacterial antibiotic sensitivity and site of infection to allow a single dosage recommendation to cover all situations. While many disease problems can be covered by routine dosage levels, special situations may require marked elevation of dosage or perhaps even allow for a reduced dosage schedule.

Routes of drug administration

The dosage form of an antimicrobial preparation determines its route of administration whereas formulation influences systemic availability of the antimicrobial agent from the dosage form (9). Antimicrobial preparations are available in a wide variety of dosage forms that include tablets, capsules, pastes, and suspensions for oral and intra-uterine administration; sterile solutions and suspensions for injections; ointments for ophthalmic use; and intra-mammary preparations for the local treatment of mastitis. The amount of drug in the preparation limits its use to certain species of animals, due to the wide range of their body weights. Convenience of administration and cost of the preparation are two other practical considerations that influence selection of the dosage form. The ease of administration is often a critical factor governing user compliance with instructions to administer the preparation at the recommended intervals.

Absorption is the critical factor that determines entry of an antimicrobial agent into the blood stream when an extravascular route of administration, i.e. oral, intramuscular (IM), or subcutaneous (SC) injection is used. Absorption, the extent of which depends mainly on the physicochemical properties of the antimicrobial agent, is associated with intra-mammary or intra-uterine therapy.

Intravenous (IV) injection is often the most satisfactory route of administration for initiating therapy for animals with acute infections. Antimicrobial therapy with agents that produce a bacteriostatic effect and have relatively long half-lives (such as tetracyclines and sulfonamides) can be initiated with an IV priming dose. To avoid adverse systemic effects that may be associated with high initial concentration of drug, the parenteral solution must be injected slowly. The option to employ the IV route of administration can be limited by the lack of availability of parenteral solutions formulated appropriately for injection by this route. Because the dose is introduced directly into the blood stream, IV injection will provide therapeutic serum concentrations for a short duration than will extravascular routes that provide an adequate rate of absorption. Therefore, for maintenance of therapeutic serum concentrations, oral dosing or IM/SC injection of parenteral (prolong-release) preparations is more convenient.

The most satisfactory technique for maintaining therapeutic serum concentrations at steady-state level is to administer the drug by continuous IV infusion. The application of this technique has considerable limitations in farm animals, but on occasions, it is employed.

The IM and SC routes are by far the most frequently used extravascular parenteral routes of drug administration in farm animals. The less frequently used parenteral routes have limited application, in that they aim at directly placing high concentrations of antimicrobial agent close to the site of infection. These routes of administration include intra-articular or subconjuctival injection and intra-mammary or intra-uterine infusion. These local routes differ from the major parenteral routes in that absorption into the systemic circulation is not a prerequisite for delivery of drug to the site of action. The combined use of systemic and local delivery of drug to the site of infection represents the optimum approach to treatment of conditions where the infection site may be relatively inaccessible, such as in a cow with mastitis (9).

Absorption of antimicrobial agents from the IM and SC sites of injection takes place by passive diffusion, similar to that from the gastro-intestinal tract, as well as by bulk flow through intercellular pores in the capillary endothelial membrane. Factors that influence absorption include the physicochemical properties of the drug, that govern its passage across the membrane separating the absorption site from the blood, the pH of the solution at the absorption site, and the local blood flow. Because most antimicrobial agents are weak organic acids or bases, the physicochemical properties that affect their membrane penetrative capacity are the degree of ionization and lipid-solubility. The less ionized and more lipid-soluble the drug, the greater will be the rate of absorption by passive diffusion. In addition to and often overriding the physicochemical properties of the drug is the influence of formulation of the preparation (dosage form) on the bio-availability.

Age or body weight can affect the systemic availability of many antimicrobial agents. In the physically smaller animal (sheep and pig) the peak serum concentration of a drug is usually higher and is followed by a rapid decline compared with a lower peak and a slower decline of the antibiotic in serum of the larger animal (cow and horse). The limited experimental data appear to indicate that the extent of systemic availability of IM-administered antibiotics can vary as widely between different sites as between IM and SC sites. A corollary to this observation is that the location of the extravascular injection site should be well-defined when determining the systemic availability of parenteral preparations (9).

A prolonged-release dosage form is one that not only contains more drug than a conventional dosage form but releases its drug content more slowly than the conventional preparation. The objective of treatment with a prolonged release antimicrobial preparation is to achieve a situation in which the duration of antibacterial effect is controlled by the rate of drug release from the dosage form rather than by the disposition kinetics of the drug. The convenience of a single administration is an obvious advantage. An important feature in the design of prolonged-release dosage forms is that the rate of release be adequate to maintain effective serum drug concentrations. Another requirement is that the formulation of parenteral preparations be such that their IM injection does not cause tissue damage with persistence of residual concentrations at the injection site.

Sporadic clinical reports, without the support of data from controlled studies, repeatedly indicate the effectiveness of intratracheal administration of parenteral antimicrobial preparations in the treatment of tracheobronchitis and pneumonia in cattle. The expectation when using this route of administration is that a greater therapeutic effect will be achieved when the drug is placed as close to the infection site as possible, rather than relying on the systemic circulation for drug delivery.

The majority of oral preparations are solid dosage forms. These include tablets and capsules for administration to small farm animals, pastes for horses, and a variety of prolonged-release products for administration to cattle. The drug in solid dosage form must dissolve before it can be absorbed. The dissolution rate depends in part on the physicochemical properties of the drug and partly on the manufacturing process. The inert ingredients of the dosage form can have a profound effect on dissolution of the active ingredient and thereby control its rate of absorption. Dissolution is often the major underlying source of variation in the absorption of a drug from different oral preparations, and this process can even influence the effectiveness of therapy.

Even though a drug may have the combination of physicochemical properties that are favourable for absorption, it may still have low systemic availability when administered orally. The drug may be unstable in gastro-intestinal fluids (such as penicillin G) or be metabolized. Metabolism can be mediated by intestinal microflora or epithelial enzymes or can occur in the liver preceding entry of the drug into the systemic circulation. The importance of the first-pass effect does not appear to have been determined for antimicrobial agents in farm animals, but presumably would apply only to lipophilic agents that are extensively metabolized (such as chloramphenicol, clindamycin, metronidazole, trimethoprim, and the antibacterial quinolones).

The ruminal microflora can hydrolize esters and have been shown to inactivate chloramphenicol by reductive reactions. In calves less than one-week old, chloramphenicol is well absorbed when administered as an oral solution. The systemic availability of the antibiotic decreases with ruminal development. Similar observations were made after oral ampicillin, amoxycillin and cephalexin therapy in young calves. Trimethoprim is extensively metabolized in the liver (oxydation followed by conjugation reactions) and may undergo some metabolism in the rumen. The higher systemic availability of trimethoprim in the newborn calf and kid can be attributed to lower metabolic activity with lesser first-pass effect in the neonatal animal. Although some antimicrobial agents can be metabolized in the rumen, prolonged oral dosing with these or other agents has the potential to disturb activity of the ruminal microflora (9). Thus, knowledge of the bio-availability and disposition kinetics of the antimicrobial agent is required for optimal dosage with the preparation selected. This information can only be obtained from well-designed pharmacokinetic studies in the target species of farm animals.

Types of antimicrobial agents

Penicillins. This group includes penicillin G (benzyl-penicillin), penicillin VK (phenoxymethyl-penicillin), the isoxazolyl penicillins oxacillin, cloxacillin, dicloxacillin and nafcillin, the amino-penicillins ampicillin, hetacillin and amoxycillin, the carboxy-penicillin carbenicillin, and the thienyl-penicillin ticarcillin.

These antibiotics are bactericidal via inhibition of synthesis of cell wall material necessary for maintenance of cellular integrity. The spectrum of action is quite broad for the group as a whole; however, specific penicillins may have a limited range of efficacy. Penicillin G is not only one of the oldest antibiotics, but remains one of the most useful. It is limited by its poor tissue distribution and its low sensitivity for Gram-negative bacteria. These limitations can often be overcome, however, by increasing the dosage since both cost and toxicity are low. Increasing the dose to increase tissue levels is best accomplished using either the water-soluble Na and K salts IV or the Na salt IM. By these routes of administration the increases in serum or tissue concentrations are nearly proportional to increases in dose. Dosage of procaine penicillin G must be increased markedly to produce a useful increase in serum or tissue level while benzathine penicillin G can only be used to provide prolonged low levels regardless of the dose. The isoxazolyl penicillins are used primarily for the intra-mammary treatment of mastitis due to penicillinase-producing staphylococci.

The amphoteric amino-penicillins have become popular because of their efficacy against many Gram-negative pathogens associated with neonatal infections, such as enteritis and pneumonia. Although ampicillin is a very effetive drug, it erratic oral absorption in preruminants is an important limiting factor. With oral use, the dosage should be increased and administered several hours prior to or after feeding. Hetacillin is not appreciably better than ampicillin in the above respects. Amoxycillin, a very similar drug to ampicillin, does not share these restrictions as it is well absorbed in the presence of food. Sodium salt preparations of ampicillin are available for short duration, high serum levels while the trihydrate forms are analogous to procaine penicillin G in producing sustained low serum and tissue levels.

Penicillins available with specific efficacy against Pseudomonas spp. include carbenicillin and ticarcillin. Both are very effective but require high dosage (50 mg/kg). They can also be used concurrently with aminoglycosides but should be injected separately. Cost is a limiting factor in the use of these drugs.

Cephalosporins. These beta-lactam antibiotics share many features with the penicillins including mechanism, spectrum of action, distribution ans toxicity potential. At the present time, the cephalosporins are classified into three groups, designated as generations.

First-generation cephalosporins, introduced into human medicine in the 1960's and 1970's, are basically similar in antibacterial activity and differ mainly in their pharmacokinetic properties. These include all of the currently available orally active cephalosporins, and are relatively susceptible to beta-lactamase, active against most Gram-positive bacteria and have a limited spectrum of activity against the Gram-negative organisms.

Second-generation cephalosporins, initially introduced in the late 1970's, tend to be more resistant to beta-lactamase and more active against a broader spectrum of Gram-negative bacteria. Although their activity against Gram-positive bacteria is often thought to be less than the first-generation compounds, this is usually in reference to the penicillin-resistant staphylococci.

Third-generation cephalosporins were introduced in the early 1980's. They are more active against many of the Gram-negative organisms, including Pseudomonas spp., often at the expense of diminished activity against Gram-positive bacteria, particularly S. aureus. Some third generation cephalosporins have long half-lives as well as good penetration of CSF and peritoneal fluid.

The cephalosporins are not widely used in veterinary medical practice due to the availability of other antibiotics that are effective against the common animal pathogens, less expensive on a treatment regimen basis, and approved for use in animals. At the present time, only a single first-generation cephalosporin, cephapirin, is approved for use in food animals in the USA. Available as an intra-mammary infusion preparation, cephapirin is used in the treatment of mastitis in lactating and non-lactating cows. The first-generation cephalosporins cephalexin, cephoxazole, cephalonium, cephacetrile and cefuroxime are approved in several European countries as intra-mammary infusion products for the treatment of mastitis in cows. Cephalexin is also used parenterally for the treatment of neonatal infections in calves and for bovine mastitis. In most cases, the cephalosporins are not the preferred drug, but rather used in infections caused by organisms resistant to other antibiotics. However, there is a trend to use the cephalosporins for presurgical prophylaxis, especially in certain orthopedic procedures. The cephalosporin antibiotics are among several classes of compounds currently being examined in a search for new therapeutic antibacterials for use in veterinary medicine, with primary emphasis on products for food animals (10).

Aminoglycosides (aminocyclitols). These antibiotics are valuable therapeutic agents and among the oldest known antibacterial agents for use in farm animals. They include streptomycin, neomycin, kanamycin, gentamycin, spectinomycin, and the recently introduced amikacin and apramycin. All are rapidly bactericidal and their activity involves uptake of the antibiotic by bacteria followed by binding to bacterial ribosomes and inhibition of protein synthesis. Their spectrum of activity covers most Gram-negative bacteria, as well as staphylococci but they have relatively poor activity against streptococci and no useful activity against anaerobic bacteria or fungi. Bacteria acquire resistance to aminoglycosides by (i) mutation of the organism leading to altered ribosomes that no longer bind the drug, (ii) by reduced permeability of the bacterium to the drug, or (iii) by bacterial enzymes that inactivate the drug.

All aminoglycoside antibiotics are small, basic water-soluble molecules that form stable salts. None is absorbed well from the alimentary tract or when applied topically, and therefore, must be administered parenterally for systemic use. In human beings, there is a higher risk of toxicosis when aminoglycoside agents are administered by IV bolus injection or continuous IV infusion. The margin between therapeutic and toxic concentrations for all members of this group is not as great as that with the penicillins or macrolides. The two problems occurring less frequently but of great concern are neuromuscular blockage and cardiovascular depression. Ototoxicity is manifested by damage to the 8th cranial nerve which include auditory and vestibular dysfunction. Studies of the acoustical effects of aminoglycoside antibiotics in domestic animals have been limited because of difficulties in determining hearing loss in animals. Nephrotoxicity is of great potential importance because approximately 90% of drug is eliminated by renal filtration. Any failure in renal filtration will result in an excessively high serum concentration of aminoglycoside which in turn will result in further renal injury. Aminoglycosides accumulate in renal parenchyma, mainly in the cortex, in concentrations considerably greaters than those in serum.

Streptomycin is widely used generally in combination with penicillin for treatment of cattle with shipping fever, mastitis or after surgery and trauma.

Neomycin is commonly used in combination with other drugs. Parenterally, neomycin is quite nephrotoxic. It is most often used topically in animals with infectious diseases of the eye and external ear or contaminated wounds. Neomycin is also available alone or in combination with other drugs for the treatment of enteric infections and for the intra-mammary treatment of mastitis in cows.

Kanamycin is unapproved in the USA for use in food animals but in many other countries it is used for the treatment of cattle with respiratory tract diseases, mastitis, and other infectious diseases.

Gentamicin is indicated for control of bacterial infections of the uterus in horses and cattle and as an aid to improving conception. Treatment is given by intra-uterine infusion of 2 g mixed with 200 ml sterile saline daily for 3 days. Gentamicin is also indicated for the treatment of pigs with colibacillosis or swine dysentry IM or orally as well as drinking water administration. Although unapproved in the USA, gentamicin has been used in cattle by intra-mammary infusion for treatment of mastitis, by intra-uterine infusion for treatment of metritis, and parenterally for treatment of respiratory tract infections (11).

Amikacin is indicated for the treatment of genital tract infections in the mare by intra-uterine infusion.

Apramycin is unapproved for use in the USA for food animals but in many European countries it is widely used for the same indications as neomycin. Apramycin is effective in vitro against neomycin- and streptomycin-resistant Gram-negative bacteria associated with diseases of new born calves.

The future development of aminoglycosides for use in veterinary medicine will depend on two main factors. The first is the cost of producing them as the synthetic process is expensive. The second is depdendent on discovering an aminoglycoside that does not accumulate and remain in kidney tissue for prolonged periods, resulting in a shorter withdrawal period for food producing animals (11).

Macrolides. This group includes erythromycin, tylosin, oleandomycin and spiramycin. These antibiotics are bacteriostatic and are active against Gram-positive bacteria, including penicillin G-resistant staphylococci, and mycoplasma. They are lipophillic weak bases and can achieve excellent tissue penetration and relatively long tissue life. In such tissues as lung and mammary gland, drug concentrations may be 3 to 4 times serum levels. Oral absorption is variable with erythromycin and may be reduced by the presence of feed for some preparations (6). Absorption from IM injection site is slow and because of the wide tissue distribution high serum levels are difficult to attain. They are used parenterally and orally for the treatment of respiratory infections, particularly those associated with Mycoplasma spp. and for the intra-mammary treatment of bovine mastitis.

Tetracyclines. Oxytetracycline is widely used in clinical practice against a broad array of pathogens although its efficacy against some Gram-negative bacteria has declined in recent years. The extensive tissue distribution of this group is of particular value in the treatment of respiratory tract infections. Although all the tetracyclines are well distributed to respiratory tissues, including the sinuses, doxycycline appears to accumulate in bronchial fluids and may have particular value in chronic bronchial infections. Oral absorption is good in monogastrics, but questionable in ruminants. Although systemic effects are attainable by oral administration in ruminants, high serum levels are best achieved by IV administration. The recently introduced long-acting (LA) formulations of oxytetracycline have gained great popularity. They are used at a relatively high dose (20 mg/kg) and serum levels sufficient to inhibit the growth of susceptible pathogens can be maintained for 3 days. These products are extensively used in the treatment and control of several tick-borne infections such as anaplasmosis.

Chloramphenicol. This potent bacteriostatic antibiotic remains one of the drugs of choice against many Gram-negative pathogens, although it is not approved in the USA for food animal use. It is also effective against anaerobes. Chloramphenicol is most effective when given IV. Administration by the IM route is accompanied by erratic absorption in many species. Oral administration in ruminants is not effective beyond the age of 2 to 3 weeks because of ruminal degradation. The half-life of the drug in the body is somewhat variable between species, but is generally of short duration. The drug is extensively metabolized in many species to metabolites which are inactive against bacteria. In most species frequency of administration must be 2 or 3 times daily. The drug is well distributed in the body, achieving serum concentrations or higher in many tissues. Concentrations in brain are somewhat lower than in serum but still in the effective range. This is a neutral drug so ionization is not a consideration as regards efficacy. The drug is extensively used outside the USA for the treatment of infections due to Gram-negative pathogens associated with pneumonia, peritonitis, gastro-enteritis, arthritis and mastitis.

Trimethoprim. This bacteriostatic metabolic inhibitor of folate reductase system in bacteria is available as oral and parenteral combination with sulfanumides, particularly sulfadiazine and sulfadoxine. The combination is very often bactericidal to a wide range of pathogens otherwise resistant to the sulfonamides. It is well distributed throughout the body including the reproductive organs. The need for using a relatively low dosage of the combination greatly reduces the likelyhood of toxic reactions. As of yet, this combination is not approved for use in food animals in the USA but has attained widespread acceptance elsewhere. The oral preparations are probably effective only in the preruminant calf, for others it must be given parenterally. The combination is used for the treatment of infections due to Gram-negative and Gram-positive pathogens associated with pneumonia, peritonitis, gastro-enteritis and mastitis. Some restrictive tissues (reproductive) may limit penetration of the sulfonamide component with the resultant underdosing of the trimethoprim alone which may account for some therapeutic failures (6).

Sulfonamides. This group of well recognized antibacterial drugs has long been used in veterinary medicine although in recent year their use has declined perhaps due to interest in antibiotics of more recent development. As a group, the sulfonamides have a bacteriostatic, broad spectrum of action and good tissue distribution throughout the body. The more lipid-soluble sulfonamides achieve the best tissue levels, but all are generally low in the mammary gland due to their acidic properties. Since the half-lives of most of the sulfonamides are long and oral absorption is slow, the daily dosage can usually be reduced to two-thirds or one-half of the initial dose. Of recent development are dosage forms with reduced absorption rates to prolong serum and tissue levels.

Antibiotic combinations

Any discussion of antibiotics must eventually broach the topic of combination therapy. This is a much discussed but little appreciated area because of the lack of good basic information available (12, 13). The effects of antibiotic combinations are quite specific for individual bacterial species and they may have quite diverse effects ranging between synergism and antagonism of one another when utilized against different bacteria. To fully appreciate the value of any combination, it would require testing on each bacterial species using a wide range of combination ratios. Because of this variability it is difficult to develop general guidelines. Several combinations may be quite helpful for serious illness in the weak and debilated patient particularly when a mixed bacterial population is involved. The combination may also reduce the development of resistance. In many cases, the disadvantage of increased risk of adverse drug reaction, potential antagonism between antibiotics and increased expense may be more important than the advantage of the combination.

In many therapeutic situations the drug combinations are completely misused (12). Adding another drug to a combination does not reduce the need for sound clinical judgement in therapy. Although there are many disease situations in which the use of more than one antibacterial agent may be justified, generalizations about various combinations of bactericidal or bacteriostatic antibiotics or admixtures have not proven valid. Basically, antibiotic combinations should be avoided as a common practice unless they have shown a clear increase in effectiveness as reported in the literature.

Literature cited

1. Halpin, B. "Patterns of Animal Disease"; Bailiere Tindall: London, 1975.
2. Walton, J.R. Zbl. Vet. Med. A, 1983, 30, 81-92.
3. Brander, G.C.; Ellis, P.R. "Animal and Human Health : The Control of Disease"; Baillier Tindall: London, 1976.
4. Wilson, G.S.; Miles, A. In "Toply and Wilson's Principles of Bacteriology, Virology and Immunity" 6th Edn.; Arnold: London, 1975.
5. Schwabe, C.W.; Riemann, H.P.; Franti, C.E. "Epidemiology in Veterinary Practice"; Lea Febiger: Philadelphia, 1977.
6. Burrows, G.E. Bovine Practitioner 1980, 15, 103-110.
7. Koritz, G.D. J. Amer. Vet. Med. Assoc. 1984, 185, 1072-5.
8. Powers, T.E.; Varma, K.J.; Powers, J.D. J. Amer. Vet. Med. Assoc. 1984, 185, 1062-7.
9. Baggot, J.D. J. Amer. Vet. Med. Assoc. 1984, 185, 1076-82.

10. Thomson, T.D.; Quay, J.F.; Webber, J.A. J. Amer. Vet. Med. Assoc. 1984, 185, 1109-14.
11. Benitz, A.M. J. Amer. Vet. Med. Assoc. 1984, 185, 1118-23.
12. Burrows, G.E. Bovine Practitioner 1980, 15, 99-102.
13. Stowe, C.M. J. Amer. Vet. Med. Assoc. 1985, 185, 1137-44.

RECEIVED March 3, 1986

3

Antibiotics in Treatment of Mastitis

W. D. Schultze

Milk Secretion and Mastitis Laboratory, Agricultural Research Service, U.S. Department of Agriculture, Beltsville, MD 20705

> Antibiotics have failed early expectations of chemosterilization of the mammary gland. Treatment before bacterial identification necessitates use of broad-spectrum drugs. Cure rates vary with the pathogen: low for Staphylococcus aureus, high for Streptococcus agalactiae. The most effective antibiotics against Gram-negative bacilli are not approved for U.S. use. During lactation, therapy is usually limited to clinical cases, eliminating clinical signs in 90% of cases but achieving many fewer bacteriologic cures. Mass intramammary treatment at the end of lactation is common. Higher cure rates due to higher drug concentrations and long retention in the gland, plus avoidance of milk discard are advantages. Some degree of prophylaxis is afforded against the high new infection rate in the early nonlactating period. Evidence conflicts as to increased resistance to antibiotics as a result of mastitis treatment, but has been reported for populations of staphylococci, streptococci and coliform bacteria.

Mastitis, which is defined as inflammation of the mammary gland, is the single most costly disease in American agriculture (1). Direct losses to the dairyman average $182 per cow, or in excess of $2 billion annually to the dairy industry, nearly 70% of these the result of lost milk production. In addition to the direct losses, mastitis causes significant reduction in milk quality, for both fluid consumption and for processing, and in nutritional value. It leads to antibiotic resistance problems in milk, meat and the environment, to premature culling of cattle, and to reduced sale value of young dairy stock. In mastitis problem herds, annual losses due to mastitis may exceed $300 per cow.

Mastitis is nearly always caused by bacterial infection. The introduction of benzyl penicillin for the treatment of intramammary infections (IMI) caused by Gram positive bacteria, followed by products containing other antimicrobial agents, was a major advance in

This chapter not subject to U.S. copyright.
Published 1986, American Chemical Society

mastitis control. It made possible for the first time a major reduction of the losses caused by clinical mastitis (2). It provided a practical method of eliminating Streptococcus agalactiae, the predominant pathogen at that time. Hopes soared even to the extreme of forseeing that we might be able to accomplish chemosterilization of the mammary gland, and thus eradicate bovine mastitis.

In actuality, this has been far from the case. Antibiotic therapy, although an important component of mastitis control strategy, is much less effective than could be desired. Farm advisors uniformly stress the principle that treatment must not be relied upon to redress the disease promoting effects of bad animal husbandry, unsanitary milking practices and defective milking machinery.

Mastitis is a complex of infections, caused by a variety of microorganisms with inherent differences in sensitivity to antimicrobial agents. Furthermore, sensitivity in vitro does not assure efficacy in vivo. Additionally, pathogens have the capacity to gain resistance to antibiotics, particularly under conditions of heavy and poorly controlled use.

Sensitivity of Mastitis Pathogens to Antibiotics

A senior British government veterinarian stated in 1962 (3), "When penicillin was first used in treating mastitis only 2% of the strains of staphylococci recovered from cases of mastitis were resistant to penicillin. Today the figure is over 70%." Between 1958 and 1961, resistance to penicillin (PEN) increased from 62.0% to 70.6%. Resistance to streptomycin (STR), tetracycline and chloramphenicol also increased (4). Antibiotic resistance increased for isolates of both mastitis staphylococci and streptococci in Canada between 1960 and 1967 (5). In Belgium (6), Staphylococcus aureus strains isolated from cases of bovine mastitis showed increase in PEN resistance from 38% in 1971 to 78% in 1974, but then no further increase to 1980. The resistance situation was reported to remain stable in the Federal Republic of Germany between 1962 and 1975 (7), as also in Australia between 1974 and 1979 (8) and Denmark, at a very low level, for the period 1963 to 1978 (9).

Inasmuch as selection pressure is considered responsible for development of antibiotic resistance, local differences in drug usage may explain the widely varying resistance situations (10). Great disparities have been reported within nations as well as between them, for example, in Australia (8) and Switzerland (11).

In the United States, it is the common opinion (based on meagre and geographically restricted data) that increasing antibiotic resistance among pathogens of bovine mastitis is not a problem (12,13), with the exception of resistance to PEN (14). A scan of reports accumulated over some 15 years (Table 1) supports the view, but also suggests a dramatic increase in resistance to STR among staphylococci. It is noteworthy that none of the drugs to which Escherichia coli is nearly always sensitive, namely gentamicin, polymyxin B or chloramphenicol, are approved for use in mastitis therapy in the U.S.

In the use of dry cow therapy (DCT) for mastitis control, we have a model situation where antibiotics are introduced into the milk compartment at high concentration and undergo slow dissipation for up to 3 weeks (21,22,23). In mass dry cow therapy (DCT), all cows in a herd are infused in all mammary quarters with an antibiotic

Table I. Proportion of Strains of Intramammary Pathogens Resistant to Antibiotics -- U.S. Data

Pathogen	State	Year	CLX	CEP	STR	GEN	NEO	NOV	PEN	TET	POB	References
Staphylococcus aureus	LA[b]	1969	--	--	9	--	1	1	6	2	36	15
"	MD[b]	1973	2	2	30	2	3	9	38	--	--	16
"	NY	1980	14	3	39	1	2	9	47	6	--	12
"	IA area	1981	6	<1	31	0	4	--	74	3	1	14
"	MD[b]	1983	7	0	61	0	14	7	61	--	75	17
Streptococcus agalactiae	IA,NY	1976	0	0	100	100	100	--	0	0	100	18
Streptococcus uberis	IA,NY	1976	5	0	100	89	100	--	0	2	97	18
"	MD[b]	1983	19	4	90	28	71	12	7	--	13	17
Streptococcus species	LA[b]	1969	--	--	42	--	4	2	2	2	48	15
"	MD[b]	1973	48	15	90	63	64	57	4	--	--	16
"	NY	1980	24	8	92	41	67	54	6	20	--	12
Escherichia coli	MD[b]	1973	100	23	53	10	12	100	100	--	--	16
"	NY	1975	100	37	31	0	14	100	100	33	--	12
"	CA,IA,MD	1977	--	40	30	0	55	--	--	85	0	19
"	NY[b]	1982	92	11	58	1	17	--	96	50	4	20
"	MD[b]	1983	95	23	55	0	27	100	100	--	0	17

[a] CLX cloxacillin, CEP cephalothin, STR dihydrostreptomycin, GEN gentamicin, NEO neomycin, NOV novobiocin, PEN penicillin, TET tetracycline, POB polymyxin B
[b] One research herd of about 180 milking cows

formulation after the last milking of the lactation. Concern about
selection for antibiotic resistance among pathogens surviving DCT
seems reasonable. Likewise, considering the entire herd, intestinal
excretion of large quantities of the drug could represent a continual
selective pressure on the fecal coliform flora and thus on the environmental flora. An investigation of the latter situation (24)
showed that DCT with large doses of PEN and STR had little or no
effect on drug resistance in E. coli, in either the herd or its environment.

With regard to intramammary pathogens, limited evidence showed
that most Staphylococcus epidermidis strains that were sensitive to
PEN and/or STR before administration of DCT were resistant to these
but not to other antibiotics when reisolated and tested at the time
of next calving (17). However, reisolation of the same bacterial
species is only weak evidence for survival through DCT as opposed to
reinfection. Resistance of Streptococcus agalactiae isolates from
herds practicing DCT was higher than that of isolates from herds not
using DCT (25). Oddly, resistance was increased to all 13 antibiotics tested, whether or not they were incorporated in formulations for
DCT, and resistance was not increased for the other bacterial species
examined.

Lactational Therapy

At any given time, most of the intramammary infections (IMI) in a
dairy herd are undetectable except by laboratory tests for infection,
inflammation or abnormality of milk composition. These cases are
called subclinical mastitis, in contradistinction to clinical mastitis, in which either swelling and tenderness of the udder quarter is
detectable or destabilization of the milk can be seen. In common
practice, lactating cows are treated only in case of clinical mastitis. Most products are given as intramammary infusions, in single-dose tubes after milking and in a course of two or three doses at 12
or 24 hour intervals. In acute clinical mastitis, however, intense
swelling of the udder parenchyma and blockage of the ducts may lead
to poor and uneven distribution of an infused drug. Parenteral antibiotic therapy is then frequently preferred (23).

Early detection of mastitis and immediate treatment reduces
pathologic damage and increases the likelihood of eliminating the infection. Because therapy is given without identification of the
pathogen involved, a product with a broad antibacterial spectrum is
essential (4). The desirable kinetic and other properties of an intramammary antibiotic product for treatment in lactation have been
summarized by Ziv (23).

In the U.S., unlike most nations, some antibiotic products for
mastitis therapy are available to the dairyman without a veterinary
prescription. For FDA approval of an over-the-counter intramammary
infusion product, it is required that adequate directions for use be
written so that the layman can use the drug safely and for the purposes for which it is intended. The following antibiotics are currently approved and marketed for intramammary infusion in treatment
of bovine mastitis (26):
1. OTC - cephapirin, erythromycin, novobiocin, oxytetracycline, penicillin, penicillin and novobiocin in combination, penicillin and
dihydrostreptomycin in combination.

2. R_x - hetacillin, cloxacillin, novobiocin, ampicillin, penicillin and dihydrostreptomycin in combination.
Additionally, STR, sulfadimathoxine, sulfamethazine and tylosin are available for injection.

Nearly all cases of mastitis appear to respond to antibiotic therapy because the clinical signs disappear, but this can not be equated with clearance of the pathogen from the gland. In 30 commercial dairy herds (27) 55% of IMI caused by staphylococci persisted until the end of the year of study. Only 15% were eliminated by lactational therapy of clinical mastitis, 10% were eliminated by culling of the cows and 20% recovered spontaneously. Therapeutic failure was not the major problem. When all pathogens are considered, 70% of the IMI treated were eliminated. However, only about 40% of existing IMI were detected during the year as clinical mastitis. Such results show that lactational therapy for clinical mastitis, though necessary to reduce the damage to udder quarters, is relatively ineffective in eliminating IMI (28).

Treatment of all IMI in a herd, including the subclinical, is not attempted routinely. In so-called "blitz therapy", milk samples from all lactating mammary quarters in the herd are cultured, the pathogens are tested for sensitivity to available antibiotics, and all infected quarters are treated. This is an heroic measure, applied when a sudden, rapid increase in IMI suggests that an unique, highly infectious pathogen has been introduced and threatens the herd. Alternatively, the approach is used when a herd is brought into a program aimed at eradication of a specific pathogen, usually <u>Streptococcus agalactiae,</u> or when long-term problems of milk quality threaten the dairyman's market (29).

In other circumstances, the cost of bacteriologic diagnosis is generally considered to militate against treatment of subclinical infection, with those in favor (30,31) being far outnumbered (27,32,33,34,35). However, the new infection rate of <u>S aureus</u> has been found to be related to the prevalence of <u>S. aureus</u> mastitis in the herds. Also, having one quarter infected with this pathogen doubled the risk of <u>S. aureus</u> infection in the healthy quarters (36). Furthermore, the proportion of cows contracting clinical mastitis was two to three times higher among cows with previous subclinical <u>S. aureus</u> mastitis than among previously healthy cows (37). If epidemiologic prospects were to be included in the economic analysis, conclusions as to the value of routinely treating subclinical infections might be different.

Recent work from New Zealand (38) has shown that, at least in mature cows, the reduction in milk produced by a mammary quarter affected with subclinical mastitis due to <u>S aureus</u> is compensated for by increased production in the uninfected quarters. Thus, there would be no gain in milk production from treating out such IMI. Such compensation may occur, however, only where the plane of herd nutrition is sufficiently low as to preclude full expression of milk secretory capacity, as in the full grazing husbandry of New Zealand.

<u>Dry Cow Therapy</u>

Normally, a dairy cow is milked for about 10 months after calving and then "dried off" by ceasing to milk her. Ideally, impregnation has been so timed that she will calve again close to 12 months after the previous calving. During the intervening dry period, the mammary gland undergoes profound physiologic changes that affect susceptibility to IMI (39). Early in the dry period, and again close to parturition, new infection reaches peak frequency, whereas during steady state involution new infection is at a minimum (40). To deal with the period of high infection risk just after the end of lactation, mass dry cow therapy (DCT) was conceived and validated in controlled studies by British scientists (41,42) and corroborated in the U.S. (43).

The strategy has numerous advantages. Because most IMI are subclinical, significant reduction in average duration of infection in a dairy herd requires that these as well as the clinical infections be treated. Where infection prevalence is high, as is common in U.S. herds, treating all quarters is considered less costly than sampling and culturing all quarters to detect those infected. Furthermore, the infusion of all glands with antibiotic during a period of heightened risk of new infection adds desirable prophylaxis. Treating after cessation of milking avoids the financial loss of discarded milk as well as the potential for contamination of the milk supply with antibiotic residues. Therapeutic efficacy against all pathogens tends to be significantly improved in the dry gland (13) because higher drug concentrations are permissible and the drug is not flushed from the gland twice a day at milking, and possibly because of more uniform distribution throughout udder tissue (44).

Specialized antibiotic formulations have been developed for DCT, with physicochemical properties chosen to confer prolonged retention in the mammary secretions (21,45,46). Ziv (23) has summarized the desirable kinetic and other properties of such a product. The following antibiotic formulations are presently approved by the U.S. Center for Veterinary Medicine, FDA for infusion into the dry mammary gland: erythromycin (300 mg), oxytetracycline-HCl (426 mg), benzathine cloxacillin (500 mg), cephapirin benzathine (300 mg), novobiocin (400 mg), penicillin (200,000 IU) & novobiocin (400 mg), penicillin (1 x 10^6 IU) & dihydrostreptomycin (1 g), penicillin (200,000 IU) & dihydrostreptomycin (300 mg), and procaine penicillin G (100,000 IU) (26).

Varying estimates of therapeutic success from use of dry cow formulations have been reported (Table II). Correction for spontaneous cure rate in an appropriate control group is necessary to preclude serious overestimation of drug efficacy.

Mass DCT is a popular and commonly recommended strategy in the U.S., the U.K., Australia, Ireland, the Federal Republic of Germany, France, the Netherlands, South Africa and Israel (54). Antimicrobial treatment at drying off is rarely practiced in Austria, Czechoslovakia, Hungary, Spain, Japan, Norway and Poland. New Zealand and most of the Scandinavian countries favor selective DCT, in which only those cows receive treatment who have either a history of clinical mastitis during the preceding lactation or current signs of infection (54). It has been suggested that as mastitis control using the strategies common among the English-speaking countries reduces disease prevalence we must rethink the question of mass versus selective therapy (55).

Selective Dry Cow Therapy. Two criteria are critical to the success of a regimen for selective DCT: the ability to detect and thus

Table II. Efficacy of Dry Cow Therapy Against Intramammary Infections

Antibiotics in formulation	Staphylococcus aureus	Streptococcus agalactiae	Streptococcus other	Coliform bacteria	References
		%[a]			
Procaine penicillin G (1 x 10⁶ IU); dihydrostreptomycin-SO_4 (1 g)	87	97	90	--	41
Benzathine penicillin G (200,000 IU); dihydrostreptomycin-SO_4 (0.4 g)	76	-------- combined 97 --------		--	46
Benzathine cloxacillin (1 g)	84			--	47
Benzathine cloxacillin (0.5 g)	74[b]	91[b]	59[b]	11[b]	48
Benzathine cloxacillin (0.5 g)	79[b]	90[b]	56[b,c]	--	49
Neomycin-SO_4 (0.5 g)	62	65	75	89	48
Neomycin-SO_4 (0.5 g); benzathine penicillin V (325,000 IU)	77[b]	90[b]	100[b,c]	--	49
Procaine penicillin G (500,000 IU); novobiocin (0.6 g)	35[b]	--	45[b]	31[b]	50
Procaine penicillin G (200,000 IU); novobiocin (0.4 g)	61	--	--	--	51
Novobiocin (0.4 g)	34[b]	88[b]	67[b]	--	52

[a] Percent of infected quarters rendered noninfected
[b] Percentage computed by correcting for author's reported spontaneous cure rate
[c] Streptococcus uberis only

select for treatment a high proportion of cows with IMI present at drying off, and achievement of a degree of prophylaxis not greatly inferior to that afforded by mass DCT. Studies of efficiency of detection have not been encouraging. Selection for treatment of individual quarters according to their strong reaction in the Whiteside test (a rough measure of inflammation of the gland) (56) detected only 39% of infected quarters and predictably would have permitted 80% of all staphylococcal infections to persist into the next lactation. Treating all quarters of cows which had had clinical mastitis during the previous lactation (57) would have missed 34% of quarters infected at drying off and 39% of those which subsequently became infected during the dry period. A comparison of selection criteria including mastitis history, somatic cell count history and current California mastitis test score, alone and in combination (58), showed predictions ranging from 50% to 92% of infected cows, but included from 49% to 80% of the noninfected cows. Selection for DCT of cows drying off with a history of mastitis treatment during lactation or with one or more quarters positive to bacteriologic culturing at drying off (17) was successful, of course, in clearing most previously infected glands. The overall result, however, was a net gain of 1.4% in infected quarters at the next calving, occasioned by the failure to control new dry period IMI among untreated cows and peripartum IMI among both groups.

Prophylactic Efficacy of Dry Cow Therapy. Prophylactic efficacy might be expected to go hand in hand with efficiency of selecting infected animals, for the new infection rate in the dry period tends to be higher among cows entering the period with at least one quarter infected (17,59). Some authorities, however, question the very existence of prophylaxis as an aspect of DCT (60). Nonetheless, one of the earliest uses of antibiotics against bovine mastitis was the prevention of "summer mastitis" (a special form of the disease not seen in the U.S.) by treating every cow at drying off (61). Field trials have demonstrated better than 90% control of this disease entity through DCT (62,63,64).

Experimental design of most studies has been inadequate to provide convincing evidence of prophylactic efficacy. Contributing to the problem, designs in which new IMI at the beginning of the dry period are lumped with new IMI at calving obscure the effects of prophylaxis. They imply an unrealistic expectation of DCT, for peripartum infection must be treated as a separate problem. It cannot be attacked merely by stretching the persistence in the gland of long-acting products for DCT. After attempting to correct for biases in selection of animals for treatment (51), prophylactic efficacy of a penicillin-novobiocin formulation was estimated at nearly 50%. Some studies in which evidence of prophylaxis against new IMI in the early dry period has been adduced have noted great differences in this regard among antibiotic formulations (65) or among species of pathogen (53). It seems reasonable to expect prophylaxis as a benefit of dry cow therapy but currently there is insufficient documentation to permit a good estimate of its magnitude.

In addition to DCT, recommended mastitis control in the U.S. includes the dipping of the cow's teats in a germicide immediately after each milking. This strategy commonly results in a lowered prevalence of IMI in a dairy herd, but also a shift in pathogen distribution. Efficacy of current mastitis control is greatest against S. aureus and Str. agalactiae, for which species cow-to-cow transmission seems of primary importance. We see an increasing number of dairy herds in which the mastitis problem stems chiefly from exposure of teat ends between milkings, to pathogens originating in the cow's environment: streptococci other than Str. agalactiae and Gram-negative bacilli members of the coliform group (66). For such herds, restricted application of DCT would seem reasonable if the sacrifice of potential prophylaxis in the early dry period were not too great.

Antibiotic Activity and Phagocytosis

Sensitivity of mastitis pathogens to an antibiotic in vitro merely indicates potential therapeutic efficacy. The data from clinical trials reflect a less encouraging reality, in which both pathogen and host characteristics influence the outcome (67). Some pathogens are highly tissue-invasive. Once sequestered and metabolically inactive within infection foci they are unaffected by antibiotics that act by disruption of cell wall synthesis, such as penicillins and cephalosporins.

The aim of antimicrobial therapy is to kill or temporarily inactivate a sufficient proportion of the population of invading bacteria to permit host defense mechanisms to accomplish sterilization of the affected tissue (67). Phagocytosis of cells of the pathogen by several classes of blood-derived leukocytes is a critical element in the process. However, intracellular survival within phagocytic cells can be a significant contributor to failure of antibiotic therapy (68). At least in the case of Staphylococcus aureus, phagocytosis is not always followed by killing, and can indeed protect the engulfed bacteria from exposure to cloxacillin for up to 4 days.

Furthermore, antibiotics and formulation vehicles used in intramammary infusion therapy against mastitis can have a deleterious effect on the viability and phagocytic activity of neutrophilic leukocytes isolated from bovine milk. In an in vitro assay for phagocytosis of ^{32}P-labeled S. aureus, the percentage of phagocytosis was significantly reduced by addition to the incubation mixture of tiamulin, nitrofurantoin, rifampin, chloramphenicol or amikacin in quantities reflective of their concentration in milk 6 h after injection into a mammary gland (69). Also, gentamicin, tetracycline, and novobiocin-penicillin were inhibitory at a concentration similar to that in milk immediately after injection. Incubation with chloramphenicol, novobiocin-penicillin or tiamulin also affects overall neutrophil viability, as measured by exclusion of trypan blue dye from the cell (70). Disruption of the morphology and function of bovine milk neutrophils was produced in vivo by intramammary infusion of tetracycline, gentamicin or chloramphenicol (71).

Coda

Nowadays, one stated objective of much of the more imaginative mastitis research is the reduction in our dependence on antibiotics and other exogenous chemicals to control bovine mastitis. Achievement of this goal is nowhere in sight. And so, we are left dependent upon antimicrobial therapy, despite its many limitations, as a major element in control strategy for bovine mastitis.

Literature Cited

1. Jasper, D. E.; McDonald, J. S.; Mochrie, R. D.; Philpot, W. N.; Farnsworth, R. J.; Spencer, S. B. Proc. 21st Annu. Mtg. Nat. Mastitis Coun., 1982, pp. 182-4.
2. IDF Group of Experts on Mastitis. "Principles of Mastitis Control"; International Dairy Federation Doc. 76: Brussels, 1973; p. 67.
3. Wilson, C. D. J. Soc. Dairy Technol. 1962, 15, 21-7.
4. Wilson, C. D. Vet. Rec. 1961, 73, 1019-24.
5. Greenfield, J.; Bankier, J. C. Can. J. comp. Med. 1969, 33, 39-43.
6. Devriese, L. A. Ann. Rech. Vet. 1980, 11, 399-408.
7. Weigt, U.; Bleckmann, E. Dtsch. Tierärztl. Wschr. 1977, 84, 234-5.
8. Frost, A. J.; O'Boyle, D. Aust. vet. J. 1981, 57, 262-7.
9. Madsen, J. A. Nord. Vet-Med. 1978, 30, 434-6.
10. Finland, M. J. Inf. Dis. 1970, 122, 419-31.
11. Schifferli, D.; Schällibaum, M.; Nicolet, J. Schweiz. Arch. Tierheilk. 1984, 126, 83-90.
12. Davidson, J. N. Proc. 19th Annu. Mtg. Nat. Mastitis Coun., 1980, pp. 181-5.
13. Natzke, R. P. Proc. 21st Annu. Mtg. Nat. Mastitis Coun., 1982, pp. 125-33.
14. McDonald, J. S.; Anderson, A. J. Cornell Vet. 1981, 71, 391-6.
15. Philpot, W. N. J. Dairy Sci. 1969, 52, 708-13.
16. Schultze, W. D. Proc. 26th Annu. Mtg. Northeastern Mastitis Conf. 1973, pp. 67-74.
17. Schultze, W. D. J. Dairy Sci. 1983, 66, 892-903.
18. McDonald, J. S.; McDonald, T. J.; Stark, D.R. Am. J. Vet. Res. 1976, 37, 1185-8.
19. McDonald, J. S.; McDonald, T. J.; Anderson, A. J. Am. J. Vet. Res. 1977, 38, 1503-7.
20. Davidson, J. N. J. Am. Vet. Med. Assoc. 1982, 180, 153-5.
21. Ziv, G.; Saran-Rosenzuaig, A.; Risenberg, R. Zbl. Vet. Med. B 1973, 20, 415-24.
22. Ziv, G.; Gordin, S.; Bechar, G.; Bernstein, S. Br. vet. J. 1976, 132, 318-22.
23. Ziv, G. Vet.Med./S.A.C. 1980, 75, 657-70.
24. Rollins, L.D.; Pocurull, D. W.; Mercer, H. D.; Natzke, R. P.; Postle, D. S. J. Dairy Sci. 1974, 57, 944-50.
25. Berghash, S. R.; Davidson, J. N.; Armstrong, J. C.; Dunny, G. M. Antimicrobial Agents Chemotherapy 1983, 24, 771-6.
26. Anonymous. "National Drug Withdrawal Guide for Dairymen"; National Milk Producers Federation: Arlington, 1982.
27. Griffin, T. K.; Dodd, F. H.; Bramley, A. J. Proc. Br. Cattle Vet. Assoc. 1981-82, 1982, pp. 137-52.
28. Bramley, A. J.; Dodd, F. H. J. Dairy Res. 1984, 51, 481-512.
29. Nicolet, J.; Schällibaum, M.; Schifferli, D.; Schweizer, R. Schweiz. Arch. Tierheilk. 1983, 125, 31-43.
30. Olsen, S. J. In "Proc. IDF Seminar on Mastitis Control 1975"; International Dairy Federation Doc. 85: Brussels, 1975; pp. 410-41.

31. Klastrup, O. In "Proc. Symposium on Mastitis Therapy, Copenhagen"; Novo Industri A/S: Bagsvaerd, Copenhagen, 1982; pp. 1-7.
32. Senze, A.; Jakubowski, S. Zeszyt. nauk. wyzsz. Szkol. roln., Wroclaw 1957, No. 10 (Weterynaria III), 135-49 (summary in Ger.)
33. Morris, R. S. Aust. vet. J. 1973, 49, 153-6.
34. Plommet, M.; Le Loudec, C. In "Proc. IDF Seminar on Mastitis Control 1975"; International Dairy Federation Doc. 85: Brussels, 1975; pp. 265-81.
35. McDermott, M. P.; Erb, H. N.; Natzke, R. P.; Barnes, F. D.; Bray, D. J. Dairy Sci. 1983, 66, 1198-1203.
36. Bakken, G. Acta Agric. Scand. 1981, 31, 273-86.
37. Bakken, G.; Gudding, R. Acta Agric. Scand. 1982, 32, 17-22.
38. Woolford, M. W.; Williamson, J. H.; Copeman, P. J. A.; Napper, A. R.; Phillips, D. S. M.; Uljee, E. Proc. 35th Ruakura Farmers' Conf., Hamilton, N.Z., 1983, pp. 115-9.
39. Smith, K. L.; Todhunter, D. A. Proc. 21st Annu. Mtg. Nat. Mastitis Coun., 1982, pp. 87-100.
40. Eberhart, R. J. Proc. 21st Annu. Mtg. Nat. Mastitis Coun., 1982, pp. 101-11.
41. Dodd, F. H.; Westgarth, D. R.; Neave, F. K.; Kingwill, R. G. J. Dairy Sci. 1969, 52, 689-95.
42. Dodd, F. H.; Griffin, T. K. In "Proc. IDF Seminar on Mastitis Control 1975"; International Dairy Federation Doc. 85: Brussels, 1975; pp. 282-302.
43. Roberts, S. J.; Meek, A. M.; Natzke, R. P.; Guthrie, R. Proc. 19th World Vet. Cong., Mexico City, 1971, 3, 935-9.
44. Funke, H. Acta Vet. Scand. 1961, 2 (Suppl. 1), 1-88.
45. Smith, A.; Neave, F. K.; Dodd, F. H.; Jones, A.; Gore, D. N. J. Dairy Res. 1967, 34, 47-57.
46. Ziv, G.; Saran-Rocenzuaig, A.; Gluckmann, E. Zbl. Vet. Med. B 1973, 20, 425-34.
47. Bäckström, G.; Johansson, A.; Petersson, O.; Winsö, S. Svensk Veterinärtid. 1980, 32, 83-5.
48. Smith, A.; Westgarth, D. R.; Jones, M. R.; Neave, F. K.; Dodd, F. H.; Brander, G. C. Vet. Rec. 1967, 81, 504-10.
49. Postle, D. S.; Natzke, R. P. Vet.Med./S.A.C. 1974, 69, 1535-9.
50. Pankey, J. W.; Barker, R. M.; Twomey, A.; Duirs, G. N.Z. Vet. J. 1982, 30, 50-2.
51. Schultze, W. D.; Mercer, H. D. Am. J. Vet. Res. 1976, 37, 1275-9.
52. Pankey, J. W.; Barker, R. M.; Twomey, A.; Duirs, G. N.Z. Vet. J. 1982, 30, 13-5.
53. Swenson, G. H. Can. J. comp. Med. 1979, 43, 440-7.
54. IDF Group A.2 (Bovine Mastitis) "International Progress in Mastitis Control 1983"; International Dairy Federation Bull. 187: Brussels, 1985; 20 pp.
55. Schultze, W. D. Proc. 14th Annu. Mtg. Nat. Mastitis Coun., 1975, pp. 41-53.
56. Natzke, R. P. J. Dairy Sci. 1971, 54, 1895-1901.
57. Schultze, W. D.; Casman, E. A.; Lillie, J. H. J. Dairy Sci. 1974, 57, 643 (Abstr.).
58. Rindsig, R. B.; Rodewald, R. G.; Smith, A. R.; Thomsen, N. K.; Spahr, S. L. J. Dairy Sci. 1979, 62, 1335-9.
59. Neave, F. K.; Dodd, F. H.; Henriques, E. J. Dairy Res. 1950, 17, 37-49.

60. Ziv, G. In "Progress in Control of Bovine Mastitis: IDF Seminar, Kiel"; Kieler Milchwirtschaftl. Forschungsber. 1986 (In Press).
61. Wilson, C. D. In "Mastitis Control and Herd Management"; Bramley, A. J.; Dodd, F. H.; Griffin, T. K., eds.; N.I.R.D.: Reading, 1981; pp. 113-27.
62. Pearson, J. K. L. Vet. Rec. 1950, 62, 166-8.
63. Pearson, J. K. L. Vet. Rec. 1951, 63, 215-20.
64. Franke, V.; Tolle, A.; Reichmuth, J.; Beimgraben, J. In "Heifer Mastitis Seminar, Stockholm-Helsinki"; Svensk Husdjursskötsel: Eskilstuna, 1983; Chap. 2.
65. Natzke, R. P.; Everett, R. W.; Bray, D. R. J. Dairy Sci. 1975, 58, 1828-35.
66. Smith, K. L.; Todhunter, D. A.; Schoenberger, P. S. J. Dairy Sci. 1985, 68, 1531-53.
67. Craven, N.; Williams, M. R.; Anderson, J. C. Proc. 4th Int. Sympos. Antibiotics in Agric., 1984, pp. 175-92.
68. Craven, N.; Anderson, J. C. J. Dairy Res. 1984, 51, 513-23.
69. Ziv, G.; Paape, M. J.; Dulin, A. M. Am. J. Vet. Res. 1983, 44, 385-8.
70. Nickerson, S. C.; Paape, M. J.; Dulin, A. M. Am. J. Vet. Res. (In Press).
71. Nickerson, S. C.; Paape, M. J.; Dulin, A. M. J. Dairy Sci. 1984, 67 (Suppl. 1), 85 (Abstr.).

RECEIVED February 18, 1986

4
Antibiotics in Beekeeping

Robert J. Argauer

Agricultural Research Service, U.S. Department of Agriculture, Beltsville, MD 20705

A vital role insects play in the pollination of many plants, including some of our most important agricultural crops, was described in 1976 by McGregor, an apiculturist, in a handbook published by the Agricultural Research Service, United States Department of Agriculture (1). According to USDA estimations the value of crops in 1980 requiring bee pollination for seed or fruit in the United States approached $20 billion (2). Honey and beeswax produced was valued at $140 million.

In this paper we present a brief history of the use of sulfathiazole, Terramycin®, and Fumidil-B® as antimicrobials in beekeeping. Included are some results of our published research, as well as some of our new research in which we show why the precautions - stated explicitly on the current Terramycin® label to assure that honey intended for human consumption is free of trace amounts of drug residues - also implicitly apply to medicated colonies from which pollen may be collected for human consumption.

The normal honey bee colony is considered by many beekeepers as a superorganism made up of between 10,000 and 60,000 bees. A strict system of sanitation has been created in the colony in order to minimize the spread of diseases that are contagious to honey bees, Apis mellifera L. To augment this natural system, and to insure strong and healthy colonies, apiculturists, soon after antimicrobials came into general use in the 1940's, began the feeding of drugs as a preventive measure to control the spread of American foulbrood disease, caused by Bacillus larvae, and European foulbrood disease, caused by Melissococcus pluton, in honey bees.

The susceptibility of honey bee larvae to American foulbrood was described by Woodrow in 1941 (7). Farrar (8) reported in 1956 that one Bacillus larvae spore that gains entrance to a bee larva of the proper age under the right conditions may be multiplied two to three billion times in eight or nine days. He recommended that an occasional colony infected with American foulbrood should be burned. As a preventive measure, all remaining colonies should be sprayed with medicated sugar sprays or dusted with medicated powdered sugar dusts.

This chapter not subject to U.S. copyright.
Published 1986, American Chemical Society

In the United States almost all the states have laws and regulations relating to honey bees and beekeeping that are designed primarily to control the spread of bee diseases. The beekeeper consults with his state apiary inspector for state recommendations.

Sulfathiazole

Sodium sulfathiazole, though not an antibiotic, was one of the early antimicrobial drugs found effective for the control of American foulbrood. It is not effective for the control of European foulbrood. These findings were based on the research of Haseman in 1946, Johnson in 1947, Reinhardt in 1947, and Eckert in 1948 ([3-6](#)). Eckert used a colorimeter to measure sulfathiazole in a honey bee colony before and after the medicated sugar syrups were fed to and processed by the bees. He stated, "Due to the dangers of introducing even small quantitites of sulfathiazole in marketable honey the general use of this drug as a preventive measure in the control of American foulbrood is not justified at the present time." Using microbiological assay in a series of papers in the 1950's, Landerkin and Katznelson ([9](#)) confirmed that sulfa drugs remained stable for three years at 34°C in honey and sugar syrup. He found the order of stability for several drugs in sugar syrup and honey were as follows: sulfa drugs > streptomycin > tetracycline > chlortetracycline > erythromycin > oxytetracycline.

Sulfathiazole is not registered for use in the United States at the present time. Historically sulfathiazole has been used for fall feeding. If all stored food were consumed by spring the danger of contaminated harvested honey appeared remote. In 1982 ([19](#)) we developed the analytical chemical methodology based on normal phase HPLC needed to detect small amounts of sulfathiazole (Figures 1, 2) in honey and to measure the amount of sulfathiazole that may be transferred to stored honey when honey bee colonies were fed medicated sugar solutions. Figure 1 compares the separation of four sulfonamide drugs on a cyano-amino polar phase. Our ultimate goal was to determine if sodium sulfathiazole can be used in a manner that would not contaminate honey intended for human consumption. Figure 2 compares the chromatograms obtained for a sulfathiazole standard and for an extract of honey fortified with sulfathiazole. We were able to detect sulfathiazole in the brood nest honey, but not in the surplus honey (honey stored above the brood nest and available for harvest). The limit of sensitivity was 0.2 ppm. In 1983, Barry and MacEachern ([20](#)), using reverse phase HPLC, reported that of nineteen commercial honeys collected by Agriculture Canada inspectors, 8 samples contained sulfathiazole residue at levels ranging from 0.10 to 0.56 ppm.

Oxytetracycline

Registration for Use by Beekeepers. Terramycin® (oxytetracycline hydrochloride) is the only drug that is registered by the United States Food and Drug Administration for the feeding of medicated sugar syrups and powdered sugar dusts to honey bee colonies as an aid in the prevention and control of American and European foulbrood diseases. Based on approved use for feeding, given by the dusting

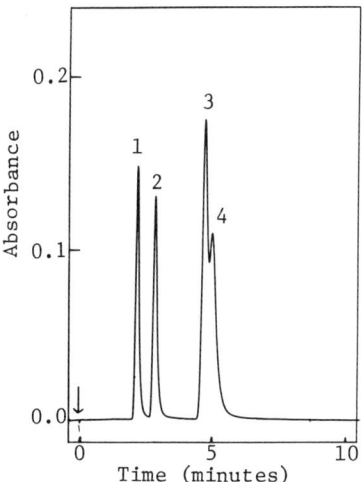

Figure 1. HPLC separation of four sulfonamide drugs on a $CN-NH_2$ bonded polar phase (1) Sulfadiazine; (2) sulfapyridine; (3) sulfanilamide; (4) sulfathiazole. Mobile phase: 95% methylene chloride-5% methanol; flow rate 1 ml/min. Detection: 254 nm. Amount injected: 0.2 µg each (as the free acids obtained from Sigma Chemical Co.).

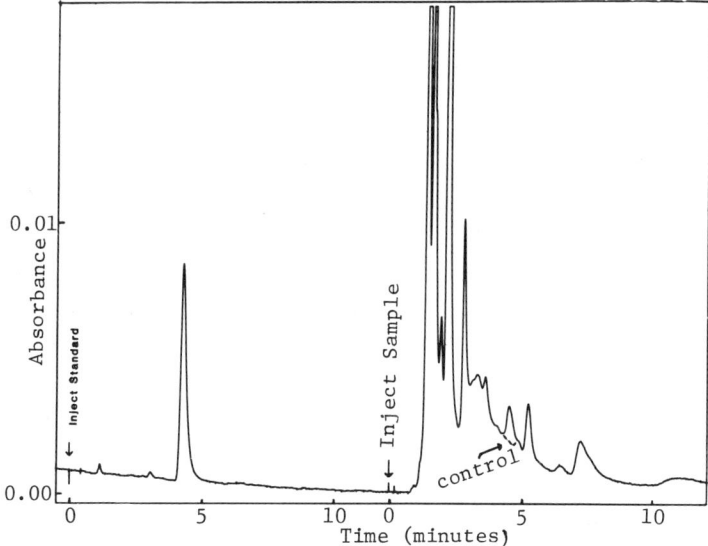

Figure 2. HPLC chromatograms obtained for sulfathiazole standard compared with a honey control and honey fortified at 1.0 ppm (80% recovery). Mobile phase: 95% methylene chloride-5% methanol; flow rate 1.5 ml/min; 0.2 µg of sulfathiazole injected as standard; extract injected equivalent to 40 mg of honey.

and syrup directions printed on the label (Table I), each colony receives 200 mg active ingredient per ounce of powdered sugar sprinkled on the ends of the frames, or 50 micrograms active ingredient in each milliliter of sugar syrup fed either by using feeders or by filling the brood combs to cause gourging. To avoid contamination of marketable honey by trace amounts of oxytetracycline, all medicated sugar dusts and syrup treatments of honey bee colonies that occur in the spring and/or fall are terminated by the apiculturist at least 4 weeks before the main honey flow begins. In addition all medicated honey or syrup stored during periods of medication in combs reserved for surplus honey is removed.

TABLE I Part of Label 60-7000-00-9 for the Use of Terramycin® Soluble Powder Distributed by Pfizer, Inc. Revised Aug. 1976

BEES

Terramycin is recommended as an aid in the prevention and control of American foul brood and European foul brood in bees. Use Terramycin as directed below.

DUSTING DIRECTIONS: Use 1 level teaspoonful (200 mg) of Terramycin Soluble Powder (TSP®) per ounce of powdered sugar per colony, or 1 lb. TM-10® (Terramycin) per 2 lbs. powdered sugar, applying 1 ounce of this mixture per colony. Apply the dust on the outer parts or ends of the frames. Usually 3 dustings at 4-5 day intervals are required in the spring and/or fall at least 4 weeks before the main honey flow to prevent contamination of marketable honey.

SYRUP DIRECTIONS: Use 1 level teapoonful (200 mg) of Terramycin Soluble Powder (TSP®) per 5 lb. jar containing 1:1 sugar syrup per colony. Dissolve Terramycin Soluble Powder in a small quantity of water before adding to syrup. Bulk feed the syrup using feeder pails or division board feeders or by filling the combs. Usually 3 applications at 4-5 day intervals are required in the spring and/or fall at least 4 weeks before the main honey flow to prevent contamination of marketable honey.

WARNING: All Terramycin medicated supplements should be fed early in the spring or fall and consumed by the bee before main honey flow begins to avoid contamination of production honey. Honey or syrup stored during medication periods in combs for surplus honey should be removed following final medication of the bee colony and must not be used for human food. Honey from bee colonies likely to be infected with foul brood should not be used for preparation of medicated syrup supplements since it may be contaminated with spores of foul brood and may result in spreading the disease.

Safe Use of Oxytetracyline. To assure honey is free from even the smallest trace of drug residue by the time it reaches the market place, researchers have developed methodologies to measure and follow the degradation of oxytetracycline by microbiological and chemical means. Recommendations for use made on the label have been based principally upon data obtained by microbiological assay that depend on the inhibition of growth of an indicator bacterium by oxytetracycline (10-12, 21). Naturally occurring antimicrobial substances that are found in honey and in bees also may give zones of inhibition which may be mistaken for activity of oxytetracycline, especially at trace residue levels. Wilson (22) in 1974, based on the residue results obtained by D. W. Clarke, Agricultural Division, Pfizer, Inc. using the Microbiological Plate Diffusion Method, Pfizer, Inc. reported that the background inhibition due to honey and/or pollen was about 0.25 ppm. In the early 1970's we developed (14) a chemical means, based upon the fluorescence of calcium-oxytetracycline complex described by Kohn (13) in 1961, to monitor the distribution of oxytetracycline in medicated colonies. We now were able to support earlier observations that were based on microbiological assay, and were able to monitor the stability of oxytetracycline in medicated diets registered for use and in several experimental medicated diets. In brief, the procedure developed involves the extraction of oxytetracycline from a trichloroacetic acid solution into ethylacetate-ethylacetoacetate, and addition of calcium chloride and ammonium hydroxide to remove the interferring fluorescent phenols and acids while the oxytetracycline remains in the organic phase as the fluorescent calcium complex. The stability of oxytetracycline in non-acidified water at brood nest temperature (34°C) is given in Figure 3. The half-life was determined to be about two days. Temperature is a variable. The stability of oxytetracycline in sugar syrup bee diets (Table II) is similar to the loss rate in water at 34°C. Oxytetracycline appears relatively stable at low temperature, and encased in experimental bee diet formulations that contain pollen, sugar, or fat (Tables III and IV).

TABLE II. Relative Stability of Oxytetracycline in Sugar Syrup Bee Diets (% Recovered)

Time (weeks)	(-9°C) Freezer	(4°C) Refrigerator	(25°C) Room	(34°C) Brood nest
0	92	92	89	90
1	90	92	70	34
2	87	90	47	14
3	90	92	28	4
7	94	86	8	3
11	90	72	3	1

TABLE III. Relative Stability of Oxytetracycline in Pollen Patty Bee Diets (% Recovered)

Time (weeks)	(-9°C) Freezer	(4°C) Refrigerator	(25°C) Room	(34°C) Brood nest
1	82	87	82	75
2	79	83	86	75
3	86	86	85	73
7	84	90	78	55
11	90	86	82	68

TABLE IV. Relative Stability of Oxytetracycline in Extender Patty Bee Diets (% Recovered)

Time (weeks)	(-9°C) Freezer	(4°C) Refrigerator	(25°C) Room	(34°C) Brood nest
1	100	98	95	98
2	96	92	91	96
3	98	97	98	100
7	97	91	95	94
11	100	94	91	97

We next applied the method to follow the degradation of oxytetracycline in syrups packed in comb cells. 700-1400 bees in small cages were medicated under controlled feeding conditions (16). Data in Table V have been "adjusted" to correct for "background fluorescence" observed in non-medicated control colonies. The amount of oxytetracycline remaining in the combs approaches the limits of sensitivity of the method 4-5 weeks after medication ends. In these experiments the highest levels in stored syrup and honey were recorded at the end of the period during which it was fed. Oxytetracycline then degrades at a rapid rate similar to that for unpacked aqueous sugar syrups. In a subsequent study we repeated the experiment using twelve isolated bee colonies maintained in large polyethylene greenhouse enclosures and fed medicated honey and medicated syrup under controlled environmental conditions (17). The rate of loss observed was similar to data in Table V down to the limit of sensitivity of the fluorescence method.

TABLE V. Relative Stability of Oxytetracycline in Packed Comb Cells (micrograms OTC/ml)

Weeks after start of treatment	Caged Bees fed medicated syrup	
	One week feeding	Two week feeding
1	124.0	113.5	-
2	30.3	2.5	71.7
3	0.0	0.2	1.4
4	-	-	-
5	-	0.0	-
6	-	0.0	-
	Caged Bees fed medicated honey	
1	165.0	177.8	-
2	30.3	9.1	182.5
3	2.7	2.6	5.9
4	-	1.4	1.6
5	-	0.0	0.2
6	-	0.0	0.0

Commercial beekeepers prefer preparations that are quick and easy to prepare and use under field conditions. We therefore compared (18) the residues in both broodnest and surplus honey after medication of outdoor free-flying colonies with medicated sugar dusts, and medicated syrup sprays that cause engorging of the nurse bees as described by Farrar (8). Figure 4 compares the amounts of oxytetracycline residues for 3 colonies, averaged for ease of symposium presentation, with a non-medicated control colony. Fluorescence readings for the control colony have been converted to oxytetracycline residue values, and have not been subtracted from the values obtained for the treated colonies. To prepare the medicated sugar dusts one teaspoon of animal soluble powder which contains about 200 mg of oxytetracycline was mixed with 28g of powdered sugar per colony per treatment. The dust was applied on the ends of the frames of the brood nest between the two brood-containing hive bodies of each of three colonies. Ten treatments were given at 4 to 5 day intervals. Medication ended after 6 weeks. Two ml of brood nest honey and 2 ml surplus honey were analyzed. The rate of loss of oxytetracycline in brood nest honey is similar to data presented earlier in Table II and Figure 3. Within 2-3 weeks after treatment oxytetracycline residues fell to levels approaching those found in the non-medicated colony. The residues found in surplus honey are relatively much lower when compared to levels in brood nest honey, and also decreased to background levels. Figure 5 compares results obtained for medicated sugar syrup sprays (18). Data for 3 colonies have been averaged for presentation. Medicated sprays sugar syrup contained 3.8g of animal soluble powder (200 mg oxytetracycline) in 1.5 liters of 50% (w/v) sucrose syrup. The combs of each of 3 colonies were sprayed with

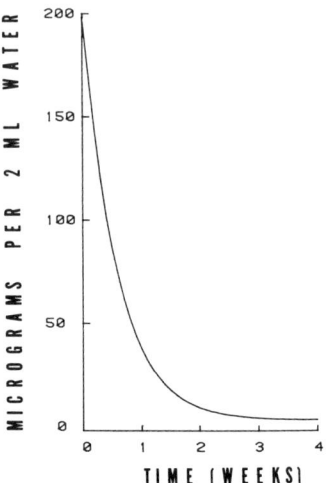

Figure 3. Degradation of oxytetracycline in water at brood nest temperature (34°C). $t\ 1/2 \simeq 2$ days.

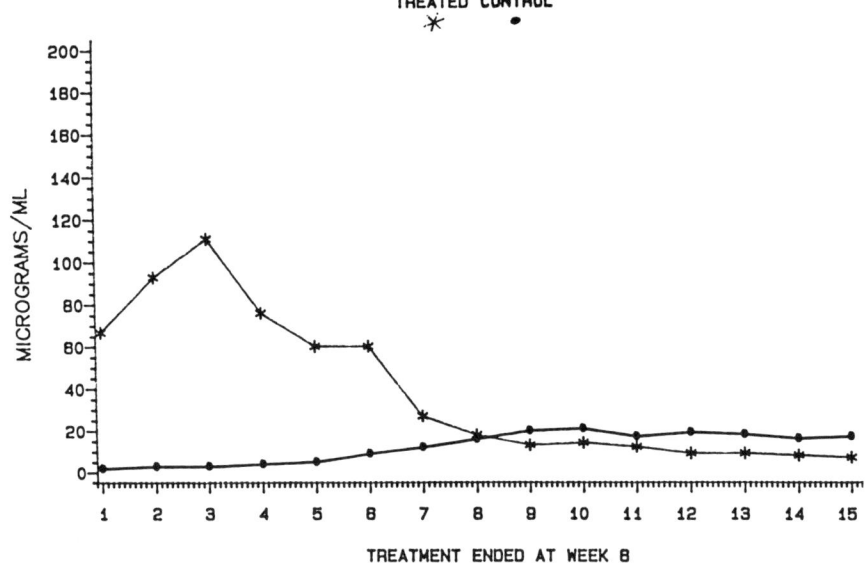

Figure 4. Oxytetracycline in brood nest honey from honey bee colonies treated with medicated sugar dusts.

750 ml of the medicated sugar syrup using a hand-held garden sprayer. Ten treatments were given at 4 to 5 day intervals. The data show no cumulative buildup of oxytetracycline residues. After the treatment ends at 6 weeks, the residues fall to levels observed in the control untreated colony.

It is clear from Figures 4 and 5 that the chemist is at the mercy of the free-flying honey bee who is free to synthesize the nectar of the gods using whatever flower it so chooses. The background fluorescence started rising on the fourth week into the experiment completely wiping out the sensitivity of the fluorescence method 3 weeks after the time the medication had ended. We suspect the increased interfering fluorescence in this experiment was caused by a flavanoid extracted from honey made from collected nectar obtained from tamarisk or athel (<u>Tamarix aphylla</u> (L.) Karst) in bloom in Arizona near the end of July. This interference was not eliminated by the extraction methodologies that we had developed earlier.

Oxytetracycline in Honey Bee Collected Pollen for Human Consumption

In recent years pollen collected in traps by beekeepers has been made available as a health food for human consumption. Commercial pollen traps are manufactured to fit inside, above or below the brood chamber, or at the entrance to the hive. Bottom traps presumably are never used to collect pollen intended for human consumption, as these traps collect dead bees and insect parts, notwithstanding the fact that medicated sugar dusts, if used, may fall from the treated frames of the brood nest chamber and possibly cause contamination. We already have demonstrated the stability of oxytetracycline when incorporated into supplemental bee diets that contain pollen (15).

Present Label Implicitly Applies to Harvested Pollen. For beekeepers who use oxytetracycline for medication, the present label (Table I) is explicit in defining the proper use and precautions that need to be followed when honey is to be harvested and marketed for human consumption. Presumably the label implicitly applies to pollen collected for human consumption as well. This does, however, pose an interesting question - if fresh pollens were collected in pollen traps placed at the hive entrance of medicated colonies before the 4 week restriction elapsed, as stated on the use label for collecting marketable honey, would the oxytetracycline be transferred by the honey bee to the pollen. To answer the question field colonies were medicated by feeding freshly prepared solutions of medicated sugar syrup for several weeks at recommended and twice recommended levels. Immediately at the end of medication, and every 3 to 4 days thereafter, pollen traps were sampled and emptied to trap samples of pollen freshly collected by the foraging bees.

The data in Figure 6 clearly show that oxytetracycline can be transferred by the bee in the field to pollen. As the pollen is being collected, the bee cements the hundreds of pollen grains together to form a pollen pellet which is returned to the hive. The amount transferred to the pollen pellet is a function of the amount of oxytetracycline that remains in the stored syrups in the colony

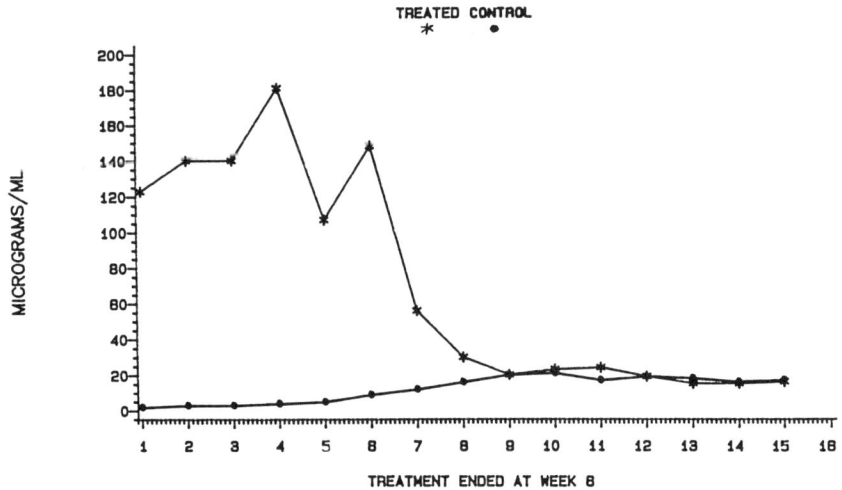

Figure 5. Oxytetracycline in brood nest honey from honey bee colonies treated with medicated sugar syrup sprays.

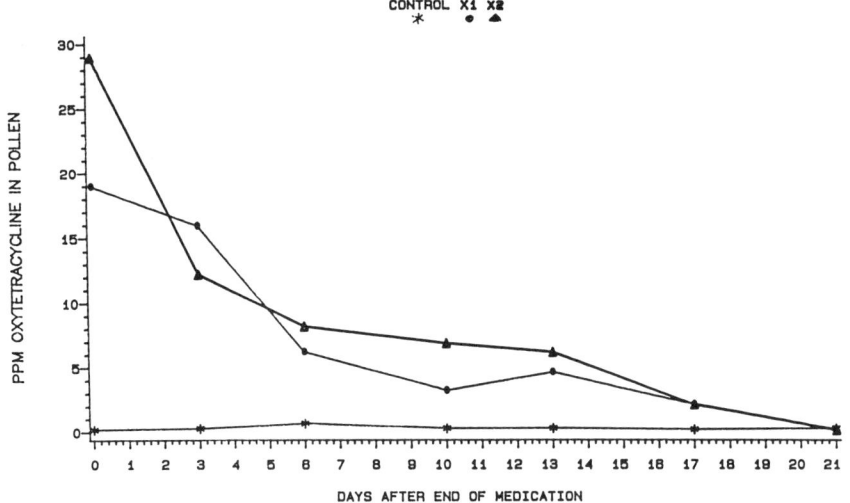

Figure 6. Oxytetracycline in bee collected pollen. Bee colonies fed medicated sucrose syrups at recommended (X1) and twice recommended levels (X2).

and on which the foraging bees feed. These data show that pollens intended for human consumption can become contaminated with trace amounts of oxytetracycline residues if precautions are not followed.

Safe and Efficient Use of Oxytetracycline - Present and Future

In this symposium paper we have attempted to provide a synopsis of some of the research that has been performed by industry and government and have emphasized some of our own published research and included new findings concerning marketable pollen, that not only supports but may help to extend the label recommendations for proper use of oxytetracycline in bee colonies. These research efforts and the work of state apiary inspectors help combat the spread of bee diseases in economically important bee colonies while helping to prevent contamination of marketable honey and pollen.

Federal Regulations. Present Federal regulations (25) limit residues of tetracyclines in edible animal tissues to tolerance limits ranging from 0.1 to 4.0 ppm (mg/kg) (26). Since tolerance levels have not been established for oxytetracycline in marketable honey or pollen, trace amounts are not permitted. Honeys and pollens are chemically complex and highly variable in their minor chemical composition, the minor chemicals being a function of the specific species of flowers the bee visits. It is precisely this freedom to forage, and the possiblity of variable backgrounds that may cause a false positive reading to be recorded when trace amounts of oxytetracycline are determined at or near the low limit of detection by either microbiological or fluorescence assay. Several methods based upon reversed phase HPLC have been proposed by Jurgens in Germany (22) and by Takeba and coworkers in Japan (23), at sensitivity levels between 0.1 and 1.0 ppm. Moats (24) has recently proposed the use of a polymeric reverse phase column to determine tetracyclines in tissues and blood serum of cattle and swine by HPLC. We expect in the near future, in collaborative work with Moats, to explore this advance in methodology in order to increase further the sensitivity for detecting oxytetracycline in honey and pollen with a high degree of confidence.

Fumidil-B

Fumidil-B® manufactured by Abbott Laboratories is the water soluble bicyclohexylammonium salt of the antibiotic fumagillin produced by the fermentation of Aspergillus fumigatus and is used world-wide for the prevention and control of Nosema apis, a disease in adult honey bees. The drug attacks the actively multiplying disease producing protozoan parasites in the gut of the adult bee.

Katznelson and Jamieson (27) first demonstrated the effectiveness of fumagillin (the antibiotic was dissolved in methanol and diluted with water) in preventing the development of nosema in caged bees. The drug's usefulness was substantiated by others (28,29). Fumagillin dissolved in ethanol solution is readily destroyed by light (30). Crystalline fumagillin exposed to light and air for one year lost 90% of its absorptivity at 351 nm (31). However when Fumidil-B is used as the source of fumagillin considerable residual nosemastatic activity is retained in stored medicated sugar syrups to permit the effective control of nosema disease (32). To protect over-wintered colonies, Fumidil-B in medicated sugar syrup is commonly fed in the fall. Colonies established from packages are fed medicated syrup as soon as they are established. Any chance of trace residues of fumagillin appearing in marketable honey from these treatments is remote since medicated syrups are not fed during the honey flow or immediately before the honey flow. Fumidil-B is inactive against most bacteria, fungi, and viruses.

Literature Cited

1. McGregor, S. E. 1977. "Insect pollination of cultivated crop plants." U.S. Department of Agriculture Handbook No. 496, 411 pp.

2. Levin, M. D. 1983. Value of Bee Pollination to U.S. Agriculture. Bull. Ent. Soc. Am. 27(4): 50-51.

3. Haseman, L. 1946. Sulfa Drugs to Control American Foulbrood. J. Econ. Entomol. 39(1): 5-7.

4. Johnson, J. P. 1947. Sulfathiazole for American foulbrood disease of honey-bees; Second Report. J. Econ. Entomol. 40: 338-43.

5. Reinhardt, J. F. 1947. The sulfathiazole cure of American foulbrood; an explanatory theory. J. Econ. Entomol. 40(1): 45-8.

6. Eckert, J. E. 1948. The use of sodium sulfathiazole in the treatment of American foulbrood disease of honey bees. J. Econ. Entomol. 41: 491-4.

7. Woodrow, A. W. 1941. Susceptibility of honeybee larvae to American foulbrood. Glean. Bee Cult. 69: 148-151, 190.

8. Farrar, C. L. 1956. Treating bee diseases. Glean. Bee Cult. 84: 207-11, 218.

9. Landerkin, G. B. and Katznelson, H. 1957. Stability of antibiotics in honey and sugar syrup as affected by temperature. Appl. Microbiol. 5: 152-154.

10. Corner, J. and Gochnauer, T. A. 1971. The persistence of tetracycline activity in medicated syrup stored by wintering honeybee colonies. J. Apic. Res. 10: 67-71.

11. Gochnauer, T. A. and Bland, S. E. 1974. Persistence of oxytetracycline activity in medicated syrup stored in honeybee colonies in late spring. J. Apic Res. 13: 153-159.

12. Rousseau, M. and Tabarly, O. 1962. L'emploi des antibiotiques en apiculture: leur action dans la ruche, leur presence dans le miel. Bull. Apic. Doc. Sci. Tech. Inf. 5: 155-176.

13. Kohn, K. W. 1961. Determination of tetracyclines by extraction of fluorescent complexes. Anal. Chem. 33: 862-866.

14. Argauer, R. J. and M. Gilliam. 1974. A fluorometric method for determining oxytetracycline in treated colonies of the honey bee, Apis mellifera. J. Invertebr. Pathol. 23: 51-4.

15. Gilliam, M. and Argauer, R. J. 1975. Stability of oxytetracycline in diets fed to honeybee colonies for disease control. J. Invert. Path. 26: 383-386.

16. Gilliam, M., Taber, S., III, and Argauer, R. J. 1978. Degradation of oxytetracycline in medicated sucrose and honey stored by caged honey bees, Apis mellifera. J. Invert. Path. 31: 128-130.

17. Gilliam, M., Taber III, S., and Argauer, R. J. 1979. Degradation of oxytetracycline in sugar syrup and honey stored by honeybee colonies. J. Apic. Res. 18: 208-11.

18. Gilliam, M. and Argauer, R. J. 1981. Oxytetracycline Residues in Surplus Honey, Brood Nest Honey, and Larvae After Medication of Colonies of Honey Bees, Apis mellifera, with Antibiotic Extender Patties, sugar Dust, and syrup Sprays. Environmental Entomology 10: 479-82.

19. Argauer, R. J., Shimanuki, H., and Knox, D. A. 1982. Determination of Sulfathiazole in Honey from Medicated Honey Bee Colonies by High-Performance Liquid Chromatography on a Cyano-Amino Polar Phase. Environmental Entomology 11: 820-23.

20. Barry, C. P., MacEachern, G. M. 1983. Reverse Phase Liquid Chromatographic Determination of Sulfathiazole Residues in Honey. J. Assoc. Off. Anal. Chem. 66: 4-7.

21. Juergens, U. 1981. High-pressure liquid chromatographic analysis of residues of drugs in honey. I. Tetracycline. Juergens, Uwe. Z. Lebensm.-Unters. Forsch., 173(5): 356-8.

22. Wilson, W. T. 1974. Residues of Oxytetracycline in Honey Stored by Apis mellifera. Environmental Entomology 3: 674-676.

23. Takeba, K., Kanzaki, M., Murakami, F., Matsumoto, M. 1984. Simplified analytical method for tetracycline residues in honey by high performance liquid chromatography. Kenkyu Nenpo - Tokyo-toritsu Eisei Kenkyusho. 35: 187-91.

24. Moats, W. A. 198 . Determination of Tetracycline Antibiotics in Tissues and Blood Serum of Cattle and Swine by High Performance Liquid Chromatography. J. Chromatog. (In Press)

25. Code of Federal Regulations (CFR), Title 21. 1979. Chlortetracycline 556.150, oxytetracycline 556.500, Tetracycline 556.720.

26. Ashworth, R. B. 1985. Assay of Tetracyclines in Tissues by HPLC. J. Assoc. Off. Anal. Chem. 68: 1013-8.

27. Katznelson, H., Jamieson, C. A. 1952. Control of Nosema Disease of Honey Bees with Fumagillin. Science 115: 70-71.

28. Gochnauer, T. A. 1953. Chemical Control of American Foulbrood and Nosema Diseases. Amer. Bee J. 93: 410-411.

29. Farrar, C. L. 1954. Fumagillin for Nosema Control in Package Bees. Amer. Bee J. 94: 52.

30. Eble, T. E., Garrett, E. R. 1954. Studies on the Stability of Fumagillin. II. J. Am. Pharm. Assoc. 43: 536-538.

31. Garrett, E. R. 1954. Studies on the Stability of Fumagillin. III. J. Am. Pharm. Assoc. 43: 539-543.

32. Furgala, B., Gochnauer, T. A. 1969. Chemotherapy of Nosema Disease. Amer. Bee J. 109: 218-219.

RECEIVED March 25, 1986

5

Antibiotics as Crop Protectants

Arun K. Misra[1]

Department of Biological Sciences, Morris Brown College, Atlanta University, Atlanta, GA 30314

> Antibiotics, the miracle drugs, have a long history of being useful in agriculture. There has been increased interest in recent years in the use of antibiotics for the control of plant diseases. Some antibiotics that are toxic for use in the treatment of human or animal diseases may be used on plants. Antibiotics have been found useful for the control of bacterial, fungal, viral, and mycoplasmal diseases of a variety of crops and ornamental plants. Drug laws of various countries differ regarding use of antibiotics as plant protectants. Concern regarding uncontrolled use of antibiotics is appropriate, but more information is needed about the effectiveness and safety of the use of antibiotics for control of plant diseases.

Antibiotics are chemicals antagonistic to life. These are generally produced by microorganisms and may be very effective against microbial pathogens(1). Using antibiotics other than in controlling diseases of humans has been called "non-medical" or "non-pharmaceutical". The use of antibiotics in food and agriculture is multifaceted(2-5) aspect of their use with plants and animals, covered in several international conferences, proceedings of which have been published(6-9). The subject of this review will be the use of antibiotics as plant protectants.

---

[1]On leave of absence from Botany Department, L. N. Mithila University, C. M. Science College, Darbahnga, Bihar, 846004, India.

Crop Protection

The use of antibiotics in plant pathology, especially for the control of plant diseases is a subject of increasing interest(10). Nearly four decades ago, in the forties, use of antibiotics for plant protection was little recognized. Antibiotics were used against plant diseases only when they were found unsuitable in human medicine(11). Later, it was found that many plant diseases particularly those caused by fungi and bacteria were effectively controlled using antibiotics(12). However, recently doubts have been expressed concerning the growing use of antibiotics(13), especially because of possible residues in vegetable products. There is, however, little evidence as to the deleterious effects of spraying antibiotics on crop plants.

Gliotoxin, isolated by Winding in 1932 from Gliocladium fimbriatum was found anatagonistic to Rhizoctonia solani, thus helpful against the root-rot of potato and tomato. Brown and Boyle in 1954(14-15) noted that penicillin was active against the crown-gall bacterium. Zaumeyer (16) found that spraying with streptomycin was effective against haloblight of beans caused by Pseudomonas phaseolicole. Zalaback(17) and Ark(18) used streptomycin to control bean blight, caused by Erwinia amylovora, under field conditions. Aureofungin was developed as a plant protectant against the fungal diseases of rice in India(19). Similarly, blasticidin has been used in rice cultivation in Japan for very long time(20).

The antibiotics used in plant protection have been more successful in controlling fungi than other types of plant pathogens. Aureofungin, cycloheximide, griseofulvin, ohyamycin and a host of others(see Table 1) have been used. Extensive reviews in this field(21-26) are available. Aureofungin is a heptaene antibiotic and is extracted from Streptomyces cinnamoseous var. terricola. It belongs to a new antibiotic group among the heptaenes(27). It is a broad spectrum fungicide, effective against a wide variety of fungi, and is systemic in activity. A golden yellow powder, it is unstable in the presence of moisture and light, and needs to be stored dry and in darkness.

A host of fungal diseases have been controlled by aureofungin(28-29). Citrus gummosis caused by Phytophthora citrophthora may be cured by 20 mg/ml spray. Control of the Diplodia rot of mangoes and the Alternaria rot of tomatoes, by this antibiotic, especially during transit and storage of fruits is noteworthy. Dipping mango fruits in 100-500 ppm of aurefungin prevents rotting for 11-20 days. Untreated fruits rot in 2-3 days. In developing countries where refrigeration is not common, this method is useful in controlling post-harvest loss.

The blast disease of rice caused by Piricularia oryzae has been shown to be controlled by a 7.5 g/hectare spray of aureofungin, four times at 12 days interval(30). Powdery mildew of apples caused by Podosphaera leucotricha can be effectively handled with aureofungin. Seed-borne infection

Table I : Some Common Antibiotics used for
Plant Protection

Antibacterial :
>Antibiotic C6, Cellocidin, Chloramphenicol, Citrinin, Erythromycin, Gramicidin, Kanamycin, Novobiocin, Penicillin, Phtobacteriomycin, Polymycin, Polymyxin, Rhizopin, Streptomycin, Agrimycin, Phytostrep, Tetracycline, and Vancomycin.

Antifungal :
>Antibiotic P3, Antibiotic P9, Antimycin, Antimvcin, Aureofungin, Blasticidin, Bulboformin, Candicidin, CRRI-antibiotic, Cycloheximide, Foliomvcin, Nvstatin, Oligomvcin, Griseofulvin, Phytoactin, Polyoxin, Tetrin, Trichothecin, Benturicidin, and Venturomycin.

Antimycoplasmal :
>Tetracycline, Erythromvcin, and Methacycline.

Antiviral :
>Actinomycin D, Antibiotic 205-2B, Blasticidin, Cycloheximide(actidione), Daunomycin DPR, Mithramycin, Mitomycin C, Pentaene G8, and Tubercidin.

---

by Helminthosporium oryzae(30) may be significantly reduce
-d by overnight soaking of paddy seeds in aureofungin solution.

Blasticidins are produced by Streptomyces grieseochro
-mogens and inhibit several species of bacteria and fungi
(31). Pseudomonas is particularly vulnerable to blasticidin
S. Piricularia oryzae causing the blast disease of rice is
widely controlled with blasticidin S in Japan. It is applied to the rice plants after infection by the fungus has
already ocurred(32), since the antibiotic affects the myce
-lial phase more than the spore phase. It would be desirable to search for spore killing antibiotics to control
soil-inhabiting microbes and to destroy the inoculum before
it infects the crop.

Numerous cases of the use of antibiotics(especially :
cycloheximide, ohyamycin, streptomycin, tetracyclines,
penicillin, griseofulvin, and polymyxin) against several
bacterial and fungal diseases are now known(33-35). In the
United States of America, Merck sells preparations of
streptomycin and Upjohn sells that of cycloheximide for
the control of the diseases of ornamental plants(R.Burg,

personal communication). Interest in the use of aureofungin is still continuing in some laboratories(36). Actidione has recently been reported to be effective against several soil fungi(37). It has also been noted that some antibioti-cs may supress <u>Verticillium dahliae</u> and protect peppers against infection and also stimulate seed germination and growth of the plants(38-39). Bacillomycin(40) has been found effective against <u>Helminthosporium turcium</u>(41), which infects several cereal crops.

Antimycin A is effective against <u>Alternaria solani</u> spores(42), karumin is effective against <u>Rhizoctonia solani</u>(43). Nikkomycin is being used to cure trees of Dutch elm disease in Hamden, Connecticut(44). It inhibits the formation of chitin and stops the mycelia of <u>Ceratocystis ulmi</u> from growing normally.

There is a long list of antibiotics that have been tried against the bacterial pathogens of plants(45-47). <u>Pseudomonas</u>, <u>Xanthomonas</u>, <u>Agrobacterium</u>, <u>Aplanobacterium</u> and other genera have been found to be inactivated by streptomycin, tetracycline, oxytetracycline, penicillin, agromycin, and vancomycin; especially in the crops of cherry, maize, bean, poplar, cotton, rice, citrus, apple, plums and several plants of horticultural importance such as geraniums(48-51)

Tomato canker caused by <u>Xanthomonas</u> can be controlled by the application of tetracycline(52-53). Streptomycin resistant strains of bacteria have been found on peach, tomato and peppers(54), and the mixture of two antibiotics has helped to stop the build-up of resistance in the patho-gens in some cases(55-56). The silvery disease of sugar-beet caused by <u>Corynebacterium</u> is insufficiently controlled by mercurial compounds, but is completely eliminated when seeds are dipped for several hours in a solution of strep-tomycin.

Most of the work with antibacterial antibiotics seem confined to Europe, India, Japan and New Zealand. Treatment of tomato seeds with antibiotics controls bacterial pathogens(57). Xanthobacidin has been said to be active against <u>Xanthomonas</u> and other species. Seed-borne bacterial tumors in tobacco may also be treated with chloramphenicol and tetracycline(58). Bacterium for crown-gall(with Ti-plasmids) can be inhibited by spraying tetracyclines on plants that are infected with <u>Agrobacterium</u>. Screening of the efficacy of antibiotics against bacterial plant pathogens is continuing(59-60). The involvement of plasmids in controlling resistance of plant pathogens to antibiotics has now been well studied(58). Caution in using antibiotics against bacterial plant pathogens is very important, to avoid resistance build-up in the environment.

The use of antibiotics for the control of plant virus diseases(61) is of interest. Several antibiotics have been tested for inhibition of replication of viral nucleic acid and/or protein synthesis within the host cell. Chloramphenicol, cycloheximide, actinomycin D and others are the most used antibiotics; and the disease caused by tobacco mosaic virus(TMV) the most treated. In most of the cases(62)the work is still at the theoretical or experimental level and the practical use of antibiotics for control of viral diseases has not been established. Principles in selecting a particular antibiotic have not been defined. Mostly a broad spectrum, relatively inexpensive, non-phytotoxic one should be selected. Those with growth stimulating activity for the host plant are preferred(63). Much work is needed in this area, but mention may be made that antibiotics are known that cure the leaf-curl disease of tomato, and also result in larger size and number of tomato fruits(60). Certain viral diseases of tobacco, potato, cucumber, tomato and other crops have been treated with antibiotics, but still many of the plant pathogens(especially viruses) causing widespread and severe damage have not been controlled successfully.

Viruses such as bromegrass mosaic, broadbean mottle, chili mosaic, cowpea yellow mosaic, cucumber mosaic, pea streak, potato virus X, soybean pod mottle, tobacco mosaic, tobacco necrosis, tobacco tumor, tomato leaf-curl and tomato spotted wilt have been treated with antibiotics such as actinomycin D, blasticidin S, actidione(cycloheximide), miharamycin A, ohyamycin, polyoxin A, pentaene G8, chloramphenicol, citrinin, daunomycin, dextromycin, formycin, kanamycin, mitomycin C, mithramycin, ribavirin and tubercidin (10,64). An antibiotic that is related to ribavirin(known in animal virology), called taizofurin has recently been tried in Sao Paulo, Brazil, against tomato spotted wilt virus(TSWV) and is said to be an efficient anti-viral drug (65). Similarly in India, DPB(code name for an antibiotic) is useful in controlling the tomato leaf-curl virus, and also increases the size of the tomato fruits(66). Cytovirin is a wide spectrum antibiotic against plant viruses, and has proved effective against the virus diseases of the crops like rice, citrus and sugarcane(Table 2).

Mycoplasma-like organisms(MLOs) and rickettsia-like organisms(RLOs) are inactivated more easily than viruses by antibiotics, since they have membranes like bacteria and are affected by antibiotics more directly during membrane biogenesis(67). Tetracycline treatment has been very effective against several MLO-diseases, especially in egg plant, sandal, mulberry dwarf, sugarcane stunt, and grassy shoot. Grapevine necrosis, hop crinkle and beet yellows are said to be caused by RLOs. Citrus greening and other similar diseases may be controlled with tetracycline, penicillin and aureofungin(68).

It is often said that when a suspected virus disease may be controlled by antibiotics(Table 3), the cause of the diseases must be mycoplasma and never a virus. This arbitrary statement segregating viruses from mycoplasma has many times been held valid, but there remain several other instances where application of antibiotics to the host plant has reduced the pathogenesis of viruses to a considerable degree(69-70).

Table II : Antibiotics Used against Plant Viruses

Viruses	Antibiotics
Bromegrass mosaic	Actinomycin, Blasticidin
Broadbean mosaic	Actidione/Cycloheximide
Chili mosaic	DPB (chemical name unknown)
Cowpea yellow mosaic	Actinomycin
Cucumber mosaic	Blasticidin
Egg plant mosaic	Actidione
Pea streak	Actidione
Potato virus X	Actinomycin, Blasticidin, Miharamycin, Ohvamycin, Polyoxin A
Soybean pod mottle	Actinomycin
Sunhemp mosaic	Pentaene G
Tobacco mosaic	Actidione, Actinomycin D, Blasticidin, Chloramphenicol, Citrinin, Daunomycin, Dextromycin, Ferrimycidin, Formycin, Imanin, Kanamycin, Laurisin, Miharamycin, Mitomycin C, Naramycin, Ohyamycin, Pentaene G8, Polyoxin A, Puromycin, Streptomycin.
Tobacco necrosis	Actidione, Chloramphenicol
Tobacco tumor	Chloramphenicol, Daunomycin, Mithramycin, Tubercidin
Tomato leaf-curl	DPB (chemical name unknown)
Tomato spotted wilt	Taizofurin

Antibiotics from higher forms of Life

Isolation and characterization of antibiotics from microorganisms has been attempted for several decades. There has recently been increasing interest in extracting antimicro-

Table III : Therapeutic drugs against Mycoplasmal Diseases of Plants

Disease	Drug	Application	Host-Plant
Dwarf	Tetracycline, chlor-, oxy-, dimethyl-, and other derivatives	root immersion foliar spray girdling	mulberry carrot tomato potato rice
Yellows	Methacycline, Chloramphenicol, Tetracycline	dipping, hydroponics, spray, infiltration	aster chrysanthemum celery tobacco
Stunt	Tetracycline	root immersion	corn
Phyllody	Doxycline	foliage dip	aster
Little-leaf	Tetracycline	foliar spray	legumes tomato
Greening	Tetracycline	sprays	citrus
Decline	Oxytetracycline	transfusion	pear trees
Spike	Tetracycline	girdling	sandal
Yellowing	Tetracycline	trunk injection	coconut palms

bial compounds from higher plants(71-73). Lichens, algae, angiosperms and various types of marine organisms are being used as sources of antimicrobial compounds(74). The emphasis is obviously on obtaining antibiotics useful in human medicine but searches may also be carried out for chemical compounds effective against plant diseases.

There are reports that plant virus inhibitors occur naturally in plants, and they could be proteins, glycoproteins, polysaccharides, phenols etc(75). Extracts of mosses, especially Sphagnum(76), algae(77) and Cassia of the family Leguminosae(78) are effective in inhibiting tobacco mosaic virus(TMV), but much more work is needed to develop viricides that may be sprayed safely and economically on crop plants in the field.

Often medicinal plants known from folk-lore are picked up and their extracts tested against known plant viruses by mixing them with the inoculum and doing half-leaf experiments. Each half of the leaf is rubbed with virus suspension, one half receives untreated virus, while on the other half virus is mixed with plant extract. Numerous plant extracts are being screened and useful compounds have been isolated. However, valid application in plant protection has not been established, although several drugs for use in human medicine have already been developed(78). Some angiosperms like Acalypha indica has been shown to be active against plant pathogenic fungi like Alternaria(79). The biomedical potential of the sea has also recently attracted considerable attention(80-81) and searches for plant protecting antibiotics are underway in the marine environment.

Legislation

Almost every country has centralized drug regulations with regard to pesticides and drugs, including antibiotics, in plants and animals. Discussions about the unwarranted use of antibiotics in human medicine and plant protection stem many times from discrepancies in the drug laws of different nations, a thorough account of which has been presented in several works(10). A very simpliefied account of the present situation regarding the use of antibiotics in plant protection reveals that there are extremes of 'no' (like in USA and Western Germany) through liberal 'yes'(as in Japan and India). Most other countries have adopted a middle path, where antibiotics are allowed in animal feed, but not in plant protection, or vice versa. Reasons for this are probably non-scientific. Much of the fear of the unwanted use of antibiotics may be removed after we have further information in the field. The USSR and West Germany regularly publish lists of chemicals that are allowed to be used as pesticides and for spraying on plants(82-83), but antibiotics do not appear in them. The agricultural uses of tetracyclines have recently been discussed. In the UK it has now been realized that a fresh look is needed at the problem of using antibiotics in agriculture (84). It is thus necessary to test more and varied antibiotics against plant pathogens, under controlled experimental conditions, before reaching a final opinion in the matter.

Growth Promotion

In addition to being used as cure against plant diseases, antibiotics may also be used as agents to stop preharvest fruit drop, or as abscission agents to collect fruits in citrus crops(85). Some antibiotics help enhance growth of the crop plants in addition to controlling their diseases (4). Hence, an ideal antibiotic that may act against pathogens, increase crop productivity and offer other desirable properties without leaving longterm residues should easily find approval with drug legislating agencies(86).

Conclusion

Antibiotics are commonly used as drugs for humans and animals particularly against bacterial infections. There has been increasing interest in the use of antibiotics for the control of plant diseases since these compounds may offer more effective and/or safer alternatives to chemicals presently used to control plant diseases. The debate over the potential biomedical consequences of antibiotics and the need to impose some kind of restraint on their usage in agriculture has become very intense lately. Caution is appropriate but the present concerns may be unfounded and excessive. The use of antibiotics has been increasing in agriculture, because of their obvious benefits. Their use seems to pose no obvious harm to the environment. It is thus better to refrain from making ill-founded arguments, and to put more effort in determining what sort of antibio-tics can be safely and effectively used in crop protection.

Acknowledgments

Dr. Luther S. Williams and Dr. Joe Johnson provided necess-ary encouragements and facilities to acomplish the task. Dr. Nipen K. Bose helped with pertinent literature on the subject. Mr. Siebrin Simon helped with improving the language of the manuscript.

Literature Cited

1. Lancini,G.; Parenti,F. "Antibiotics, An Integrated View "; Springer-Verlag : New York, 1982; p. 247.
2. Misato,T.; Yoneyama, K. In "Advances in Agricultural Mi-crobiology"; Rao,N.S.S., Ed.; Butterworths : London, 1982; p. 465.
3. Misato,T.; Ko, K.; Yamaguchi,I. Adv. Applied Microbiol. 1977, 21, 53-88.
4. Thirumalachar, M.J. In "Seed Pathology, problems and progress"; Yrinori, J.T.; Sinclair,J.B.; Mehta, Y.R.; Mohan, S.K., Ed.; IAPAR, Panama, Brazil, 1979; p. 274.
5. Navashin, S.M.; Sazykin, Yu. O. Biologischeskaya 1978 1, 19-43.
6. Anonymous; "Proc. First Int. Congr. on the Use of Antibiotics in Agriculture"; Natl. Acad. Sciences USA, Washington, D.C., 1956; #397.
7. Woodbine, M., Ed.; "Antibiotics in Agriculture"; Butterworths : London, 1962; p. 345.
8. Woodbine,M., Ed.; "Antibiotics and Antibiosis in Agriculture, with special reference to Synergism"; Butterworths : London, 1977; p. 386.
9. Woodbine,M. Ed.; "Antibiotics in Agriculture, Benefits and Malefits"; Butterworths : London, 1982, p. 367.
10. Misra,A. "Agricultural Antibiotics"; Associated Publishing Co. : New Delhi, 1980; p. 174.

11. Thirumalachar, M.J. Adv. Applied Microbiol. 1968, 10, 313-337.
12. Zaumeyer, M.J. Annu Rev. Microbiol. 1956, 12, 415-440.
13. Wen-Chieh, R.C. In "New Trends in Antibiotics, Research and Therapy"; Grassi, G.G.; Sabath, L.D., Ed.; Elsevier : Amsterdam, 1981; p. 223.
14. Woodcock, D. Chem. Brit. 1971, 7, 414-423.
15. Brown, J.C.; Boyle, A.M. Science 1954, 100, 528.
16. Zaumeyer, M.J. In "Medical Encyclopedia"; Anonymous, Ed.; Literary Books : New York, 1957; p. 251.
17. Zalaback, V. Preslia 1966, 38, 112.
18. Ark, P.A. Plant Dis. Reptr., 1958, 42, 1937-1938.
19. Thirumalachar, M.J.; Whitehead, M.D. Bull. Georgia Acad. Sci. 1971, 29, 253.
20. Heitefuss, R. "Pflanzenschutz"; Georg-Thieme : Stuttgart, 1975; p. 119.
21. Shigaeva, M.; Tulemisova, K.A. Referativnyi Zhurnal 1977, 27, 172.
22. Kurylowicz, W.; Kowszyk-Gindifer, Z. Hindustan Antibiot. Bull. 1979, 21, 115-124.
23. Dekker, J. Annu. Rev. Microbiol. 1964, 6, 91-117.
24. Babika, J. Preslia 1966, 38, 112-116.
25. Goldberg, H.S. Adv. Applied Microbiol. 1964, 6, 91-117.
26. Goodman, R.N. "Use of antibiotics in plant pathology and protection"; Amer. Soc. Microbiol. : Washington, D.C., 1967; p. 747.
27. Rahalkar, P.W.; Neergaard, P. Hindustan Antibiot. Bull. 1969, 11, 163-165.
28. Nene, Y.; Thapaliyal, P.W. "Fungicides in Plant Diseases"; Oxford & IBH : New Delhi, 1979; p. 321.
29. Agrawal, R.K.; Thirumalachar, M.J. In "Plant Disease Problems"; Raychaudhuri, S.P., Ed.; IPS : New Delhi, 1970; p. 449.
30. Thirumalachar, M.J. Indian Phytopath. 1967, 20, 270-279.
31. Yonehara, H. In "Biotechnology of Industrial Antibiotics"; Vandamme, E.J., Ed.; Marcel Dekker : New York, 1984; p. 832.
32. Misato, T. Japan Pest. Inf. 1969, 15, 18.
33. Jha, V. "Antibiotics for Plant Disease Control"; Mithila Univ. : Darbhanga, India, 1978; p. 99.
34. Vandamme, E.J. "Biotechnology of Industrial Antibiotics"; Marcel Dekker : New York, 1984; p. 13.
35. Blakeman, J.P.; Sitejniberg, A. Trans. Brit. Mycol. Soc. 1974; p. 62, 537.
36. Singh, K.P.; Chauhan, V.B.; Edward, J.C. Hindustan Antibiotic Bull. 1976, 18, 96-98.
37. Dwivedi, R.; Dwivedi, R.S. Proc. Ind. Natl. Acad. Sci. 1976; 42, 205.
38. Seredinskaya, A. F.; Sabelmikova, V.I.; Danilova, A.T.; Brun, G.A.; Osipova, R.A. Referativnyi Zhurnal, 1979, 6, 35-38.
39. Utkhade, R.S.; Gaunce, A.P. Canad. J. Botany 1983, 61, 3343-3348.
40. Esterhnizen, B.; Merwe, K.J. Mycologia 1977, 69, 975-979.

41. Subramaniyan, V. "Antibiotics, a symposium"; CSIR : New Delhi, 1958; p. 292.
42. Waggoner, P.E.; Parlange, J.Y. Phytopath. 1977, 67, 1007-1011.
43. Kanniayan, S.; Prasad, N.N. Madras Agricultural J. 1982, 69, 488.
44. Lowe, D.A.; Elander, R.P. Mycologia 1983, 75, 361-373.
45. Misra, A.; Jha, V.; Jha, S.; Sharma, B.P. In "Proc. Vth International Congress on Plant Pathogenic Bacteria"; Lozano, J.C., Ed.; CIAT : Cali, Colombia, 1982; p. 210-212.
46. Pyke, N.B.; Milne, K.S.; Neilson, H.F. N.Z. J. Exp. Agric. 1984, 12, 161-164.
47. Ellis, J.G.; Kerr, A.; Montagu, M. van Physiol. Pl. Pathol. 1979, 15, 311-319.
48. Anonymous Bull. Kyowa Fermentation Industry, Japan 1983 14, 493.
49. Fredriq, P. Protoplasmologia 1958, 4, 1-14.
50. Glasby, J.S. "Encyclopedia of Antibiotics"; John Wiley : Sussex, 1979; p. 484.
51. Knosel, D.Z. PflKrankh. PflSchutz. 1965, 72, 577-584.
52. Hardy, K. "Bacterial Plasmids"; ASM : Washington, D.C., 1981; p. 104.
53. Kruger, W. S. Afr. J. Agric. Sci. 1960, 3, 409-418.
54. Vournakis, J.N.; Elander, R.P. Science 1983, 219, 703-709.
55. Hotta, K.; Okami, Y.; Umezawa, H. J. Antibiot. 1977, 30, 1146.
56. Demain, A.L. Science 1983, 219, 709-714.
57. Trinci, A. Bull. Brit. Mycol. Soc. 1977, 11, 136-144.
58. Depicker, A.; Montagu, M. van; Schell, J. In "Genetic Engineering of Plants" Kosuge, T.; Meredith, C.P.; Hollaender, A. Ed.; Plenum Press : New York, 1983; p. 143.
59. Das, C.R.; Pal, A. Indian Phytopath. 1974, 27, 33-36.
60. Misra, A. Z. PflKrankh. PflSchutz. 1977, 84, 244-252.
61. Misra, A.; Nienhaus, F. Phytopath Z. 1977, 89, 76-81.
62. Amelia, J.C.M.; Alexandre, V.; Vincente, M. Antiviral Res. 1984, 4, 325-327.
63. Russell, A.D.; "Quensel Antibiotics : Assessment of Antibiotic Activity"; Academic Press : New York, 1983; p. 2.
64. Kluge, S.; Marcinka, K. Acta Virol. 1979, 23, 148-152.
65. De Fazio, G.; Caner, J.; Vincente, M. Arch. Virol. 1978 58, 153-156.
66. Raychaudhuri, S.P. "Plant Disease Problems"; Indian Phytopathological Society : New Delhi, 1970; p. 489.
67. Raychaudhuri, S.P.; Nariani, T.K. "Virus and Mycoplasma Diseases of Plants in India"; Oxford & IBH : New Delhi, 1979; p. 49.
68. Raychaudhuri, S.P. Eur. J. Forest Pathol. 1977, 7, 1-5.
69. Martinez, A.L. Phillipine Phytopath. 1975, 11, 58-61.
70. Liao, C.H.; Chen, T.A. Phytopath. 1981, 71, 442-445.
71. Mandava, B. "CRC Handbook of Natural Pesticides"; CRC Press : Boca Raton, 1985; p. 552.

72. Berdy, J.; Aszalos, A.; Bostian, M.; McNitt, K. "CRC Handbook of Antibiotic Compounds"; CRC Press : Boca Raton, 1982; p. 448.
73. Lewis, W.H.; Elvin-Lewis, M.P.F. "Medical Botany"; John Wiley : New York, 1977; p. 37.
74. Misra, A.; Sinha, R. In "Islamic Medicine"; Al-Awadi, A.R.A., Ed. Ministry of Public Health : Kuwait, 1981; p. 390.
75. Misra, A. Z. PflKrankh. PflSchutz. 1977, 84, 334-341.
76. Misra, A.; Sinha, R. In "Marine Algae in Pharmaceutical Sciences"; Hoppe, H. A. Ed.; Walter de Gruyter : New York, 1979; p. 237.
77. Misra, A.; Sinha, R.; Rani, P.; Sinha, M. Med. Fac. Landbouww., 1978 43, 1043.
78. Satyavati, G.V.; Raina, M.K.; Sharma, M. "Medicinal Plants of India"; ICMR : New Delhi, 1976; p.196.
79. Bhowmick, B.N.; Choudhary, B.K. Ind. Bot. Reptr. 1982, 1, 164-165.
80. Kaul, P.N.; Sinderman, C.J. "Drugs and Food from the Sea"; Univ. Oklahoma Press : Norman, 1978; p. 123.
81. Colwell, R.R. Science 1983, 222, 19-24.
82. Anonymous "Plant Protection Regulation in Germany"; Biologische Bundesanstalt : Braunschweig, 1982; p.177.
83. Anonymous "Chemical Agents for Plant Protection Registered in the USSR", 1978; Referativev Zhurnal : Moscow; p. 8.
84. Gustafson, R.; Kieser, P. In "The Tetracyclines"; Hlavka, J.; Boothe, H. Ed.; Springer-Verlag : New York, 1985; p. 405.
85. Iyenger, M.R.S. Indian Phytopath. 1979, 32, 343-351.
86. Vettorazzi, G. "International Regulatory Aspects of Pesticide Chemicals"; CRC Press : Boca Raton, 1982; p. 256.

RECEIVED May 16, 1986

Trends in the Use of Fermentation Products in Agriculture

R. W. Burg

R50G-121, Merck Institute for Therapeutic Research, Rahway, NJ 07065

By far the largest agricultural market for antibiotics is for feed additives. The bulk of this market is taken by antibiotics that are also used in human medicine. However, mounting concern over the hazards of increased resistance to antibiotics has encouraged the search for new types of antibiotics for this use. Some of these newer products are already taking an increasing share of the market. The discovery of the anticoccidial activity of monensin opened an entirely new field for the use of antibiotics in agriculture. The avermectins, a family of compounds with potent anthelmintic, insecticidal and acaricidal activity, have vividly demonstrated that fermentation products can have entirely unanticipated activities. Besides their utility in animals, they show great promise for the control of insect pests of plants. Although antibiotics have found only a limited role in the control of plant diseases, the desire to find environmentally acceptable alternatives to the chemicals currently used has prompted new research efforts to discover fermentation products for use as pesticides.

There has been a gradual evolution in the types of fermentation products that have been developed for use in agriculture. This evolution has been punctuated by several major discoveries that have served to influence future work. The history begins with the accidental discovery of a new use for an antibiotic that was already playing a major role in the treatment of human diseases. There follows a deliberate search for new antibiotics unrelated to those used in humans, the detection of a new activity for what had appeared to be a useless antibiotic, and, finally, the discovery of a family of compounds that has opened up an entirely new area for the use of fermentation products in agriculture and may well play a major role in the control of both plant and animal diseases.

0097-6156/86/0320-0061$06.00/0
© 1986 American Chemical Society

Animal Health

The market for animal health products is estimated to be over $2 billion in the U.S. and nearly as much in Western Europe. Antibiotics dominate the animal health market, and feed additives account for about 50% of that market.

A classification of the compounds used for animal health is shown in Table I. Antibiotics can be used therapeutically to treat bacterial, fungal and parasitic infections. For this purpose, they can be given in the feed, or administered orally, parenterally or topically. Antibiotics that are fed at subtherapeutic levels to improve the rate of growth and the feed efficiency are called "growth permittants". They act indirectly by a still unknown mechanism, although it seems reasonable that it is their antibacterial activity that is important, and that they must act on a subpopulation of the intestinal flora. Growth promotants act directly, through a physiological mechanism, to enhance growth; and they usually have estrogenic activity. They are administered parenterally, often in the form of an implant.

Table I. Classification of Agents Used for Animals

```
A. Therapeutic Agents
   1. Antibacterial
   2. Antifungal
   3. Antiparasitic
      a. Endoparasiticides
         (1) Anticoccidials
         (2) Anthelmintics
      b. Ectoparasiticides
         (1) Insecticides
         (2) Acaricides
B. Growth Permittants
C. Growth Promotants
```

Table II lists the fermentation products licensed in the U.S. for parenteral or topical administration to animals. Most of these are also used to treat human infections. As important as these are for animal health, of far greater economic importance are the antibiotics that are incorporated into animal feeds.

Feed Additives. Some antibiotics are also administered in the feed for the treatment of disease. These are listed in Table III. For the most part, they are used for the treatment of bacterial infections and are the same as those listed in Table II. Although these antibiotics are incorporated into the feed, their use differs from what has become known as "feed additive antibiotics" or growth permittants.

The era of feed additive antibiotics had its beginning in the late 1940's in a classic example of serendipity. Investigators at the Lederle Laboratories were searching for a more convenient source of "animal protein factor", a substance found in liver and other animal proteins that stimulated the growth of chicks fed a vegetable diet (1). [It had already been demonstrated by workers

Table II. Fermentation Products Administered Topically or Parenterally

Name	Type	EN	RE	Use UG	MA	OP
Amikacin	Semisyn. aminocyc.			+		
Ampicillin	Semisyn. penicillin	+	+			
Bacitracin*	Peptide	+				+
Cephapirin	Semisyn. cephalosp.				+	
Chlortetracycline	Tetracycline	+				
Cloxacillin	Semisyn. penicillin				+	
Dihydrostreptomycin*	Aminocyclitol	+	+	+	+	
Erythromycin	Macrolide	+	+		+	
Gentamicin	Aminocyclitol	+	+	+		
Hetacillin	Semisyn. penicillin	+	+	+	+	
Kanamycin	Aminocyclitol	+	+	+		
Lincomycin		+	+			
Neomycin	Aminocyclitol	+	+			+
Novobiocin					+	
Oxytetracycline	Tetracycline	+	+		+	+
Penicillin G	Natural penicillin	+	+	+	+	
Polymyxin B*	Peptide					+
Spectinomycin	Aminocyclitol	+	+			
Tetracycline	Tetracycline		+			
Tylosin	Macrolide	+	+			+
Griseofulvin	Grisan	Dermatophytic infections				
Ivermectin	Semisyn. avermectin	Nematodes and arthropoda				
Zeranol	Semisyn. zearalenone	Growth promotant				

*Used only in combinations

EN = Enteric RE = Respiratory tract UG = Uro-genital tract
MA = Mastitis OP = Ophthalmic

Table compiled from information obtained from (20).

at Merck and Co. that purified vitamin B_{12} could replace the protein factor (2)]. One of the materials that was tested was the dried fermentation mash of <u>Streptomyces aureofaciens</u>, the producer of chlortetracycline. The chicks grew faster and to a greater final weight than those fed a diet supplemented with liver extract, and the growth was greater than could be accounted for by the content of vitamin B_{12}. The component of the fermentation mash responsible for the stimulation of growth was identified as chlortetracycline (3), and this ability to enhance growth was quickly confirmed in turkeys and swine. The era of feed additive antibiotics was launched.

Oxytetracycline, bacitracin and penicillin were soon added to the list of antibiotics that could enhance growth and improve feed

Table III. Fermentation Products Used as Feed Additives for the Treatment of Disease

	For Use In:				Use Level
Name	Poultry	Swine	Cattle	Sheep	(g/ton)
Bacitracin	B	B	B		50- 500
Chlortetracycline	B	B	B		50- 400
Erythromycin	B				92- 185
Hygromycin B	H	H			8- 12
Lasalocid	C			C	68- 113
Lincomycin	B	B			40- 100
Monensin	C				90- 110
Neomycin	B	B	B	B	70- 140
Novobiocin	B				200- 350
Nystatin	F				50
Oxytetracycline	B	B	B	B	50- 500
Penicillin G	B	B			50- 100
Salinomycin	C				40- 60
Streptomycin*	B	B			75
Tylosin	B	B	B		100-1000
Virginiamycin		B			25- 100

*Used only in combination

B = antibacterial   C = Anticoccidial
F = antifungal   H = Anthelmintic

Table compiled from information provided in (21).

efficiency. Table IV lists the antibiotics used as growth permittants in the U.S. The levels at which these antibiotics are fed to increase the rate of gain and to improve feed efficiency are lower by a factor of 5 to 10 (cf. Table III).

There has been great concern that the feeding of low levels of antibiotics that are also used in human medicine could lead to serious human health problems. There is no question that bacteria develop resistance to these antibiotics, and that they can transfer their resistance to other bacteria, even to other species. There is also no question that antibiotic resistance has become a serious problem in human medicine. However, the extent to which the feeding of antibiotics to animals has contributed to the human health problem is still unclear and a source of great controversy.

In addition to the risks to human health, one must also consider the benefits in terms of cheaper meat and the saving of grain. In 1981, the Council for Agricultural Science and Technology estimated that it would cost consumers an additional $3.5 billion per year if the use of tetracyclines and penicillin were curtailed (4). This estimate did not consider the possibility that these antibiotics might be replaced by others offering less risk.

Table IV. Fermentation Products Used as Growth Permittants in the U.S.

Name	Poultry	Swine	Cattle	Sheep	Use Level g/ton
Bacitracin	+	+	+		4 -50
Bambermycins	+	+			1 - 4
Chlortetracycline	+	+	+	+	10 -50
Erythromycin	+	+	+		5 -18
Lincomycin	+				2 - 4
Oxytetracycline	+	+	+	+	5 -50
Penicillin G	+	+			2.4-50
Streptomycin*	+	+			12 -19
Tylosin	+	+			4 -50
Virginiamycin	+	+			5 -15
Lasalocid#			+		10 -30
Monensin#			+		5 -30
Salinomycin#			+		

* Used only in combination
\# Rumen additives
+ Increased rate of gain and improved feed efficiency

Table compiled from information provided in (21).

Because of the desire to reduce the nontherapeutic use in animals of antibiotics that are also used in human medicine, pharmaceutical companies have been searching for new types of antibiotics to be used exclusively as feed additives. Bacitracin, one of the first antibiotics to be used as a feed additive would fit this category. Two newer antibiotics, bambermycins and virginiamycin, are licensed for use in poultry and swine (Table IV). These antibiotics are unrelated to any used in human medicine and, along with lincomycin and tylosin, are taking an increasing share of the market. Other antibiotics, including enramycin F, sold in Japan, and avoparcin and tiamulin, sold in the U.K., also fall into this category (Table V).

There are some antibiotics still in development in the U.S. Merck is hard at work on efrotomycin, and Lilly has avilamycin and actaplanin (Table V). The latter is being studied not only as a growth permittant but as a means of improving milk production in dairy cattle. Unfortunately, progress has been slow and development costs are high because of the stringent requirements of the Food and Drug Administration.

Growth Promotants. Diethylstilbestrol was the major growth promotant in use for many years. It was very effective, increasing weight gain in steers by 15 to 19% and feed efficiency by up to 12%. However, it has now been banned in most countries because of its reported carcinogenicity.

The discovery of the one fermentation product that is used as a growth promotant is an interesting study in epidemiology (5). In

Table V. Feed Additives Marketed Outside the U.S. or Under Development

Name	Activity	Used in
Avoparcin	Growth permittant	Poultry, Cattle, Swine
Enramycin F	Growth permittant	Poultry, Swine
Tiamulin	Growth permittant	Swine
Actaplanin*	Growth permittant, improved milk prod.	Cattle
Avilamycin*	Growth permittant	Poultry, Swine
Efrotomycin*	Growth permittant	Poultry, Swine

*Under development

the midwestern U.S., there were reports of estrogenic effects in swine that had been fed moldy corn. The fungus Gibberella zeae was isolated from the corn, and extracts were shown to have estrogenic activity. A resorcylic acid lactone, zearalenone, was isolated and shown to be responsible for the estrogenic effects. The compound selected for commercial development was a reduction product, zearalanol or zeranol.

Zeranol does not appear to have carcinogenic activity (5). It is licensed for use as an implant pellet in beef cattle and lambs (Table II) where it has about 30 to 50 percent of the activity of diethylstibestrol (6).

Anticoccidials. A new antibiotic, monensin, discovered at the Lilly Laboratories had an uninteresting gram-positive antibacterial spectrum. However, shortly after its discovery, it was found to be cytotoxic to tumor cells in culture, and was isolated on the basis of that activity. As is often the practice in pharmaceutical research, it was submitted to other assays and was found to have anticoccidial activity in a chick assay. It was shown to control infections by the six economically important species of Eimeria that infect chickens (7). This was an exciting discovery, and there were extensive discussions between representatives of marketing and research concerning the economic feasibility of such a product. Fortunately, a dramatic increase in the fermentation yield was attained, and monensin became the dominant anticoccidial in the world. Although it has a small therapeutic index, it enjoys the unusual advantage of not succumbing to the development of resistance.

Monensin belongs to the family of polyether ionophores. These compounds consist of a series of tetrahydrofuran and tetrahydropyran rings and have a carboxyl group that forms neutral salts with alkali metal cations. Their three-dimensional structure presents a lipophilic hydrocarbon exterior with the cation encircled in the oxygen-rich interior. They probably act by transporting cations through the lipid bi-layer of cell membranes, thereby preventing the concentration of potassium by the cells. Evidence for this is that high concentrations of potassium incorporated into the medium reverse the activity of ionophores again gram-positive bacteria.

After the marketing of monensin began, there was a rush to discover more ionophores. The second ionophore to be licensed as a coccidiostat in the U.S. was X-537A, first reported by investigators at the Nutley, NJ laboratory of Hoffmann-LaRoche in 1951 (8), 16 years prior to the announced discovery of monensin. It was their misfortune not to have tested their compounds against coccidia. X-537A, now named lasalocid, differs from most of the other ionophores in its ability to complex with divalent cations. Because of its smaller size, two molecules can surround one divalent cation. Salinomycin is also licensed in the U.S. (Table III). At least two other ionophores, narasin and maduramicin, have been introduced elsewhere in the world. Narasin is a homologue of salinomycin, and maduramicin is noteworthy because it is effective at a level of 5 g/ton, only 5 to 10% of the level required for the other ionophores.

The discovery of the coccidiostat activity of monensin marks the second milestone in the history of the use of fermentation products in agriculture. Until this discovery, the emphasis had been on the search for antibiotics with antibacterial activity. It was now evident that fermentation products could be used for the control of parasitic infections.

Rumen Additives. The ionophores were found to possess a second remarkable utility. Ruminants are walking fermentation vessels that are able to convert relatively useless, high cellulose vegetation such as grass into protein. Although this is a wonderful ability, researchers, who seem never to be satisfied with nature, have long sought to improve this fermentation.

One product of the rumen fermentation, methane, is of no value to the ruminant. The major fermentation products used by the ruminant are the short-chain fatty acids, acetate, butyrate and propionate. Acetate and butyrate can be used for energy, but propionate is most useful for the synthesis of protein. If the fermentation could be shifted to reduce methane, acetate and butyrate production and to increase the propionate, the feed efficiency and growth rate could improved.

Monensin was tested in a rumen fermentation assay at the Lilly Laboratories, and it was found to produce the desired shift in the fermentation (9). Monensin has been licensed in the U.S. for use in beef cattle for improved feed efficiency, where it is administered at 5 to 30 g/ton in a complete feed. In this application, the rate of growth is not increased, but the cattle consume about 10% less food. It is also licensed for increased rate of weight gain in cattle weighing more than 400 lb. and on pasture, where it is fed in a supplement at a rate of 50 to 200 mg per head per day. Lasalocid and salinomycin have also been licensed for use in cattle.

There have been a number of reports in the last four years of studies on salinomycin as a growth permittant in swine. It has been administered at a level of 25 to 100 g/ton of feed where it gave a significant increase in weight gain and feed efficiency, quite comparable to tylosin (10) or virginiamycin (11). If these studies lead to the development of salinomyin as a growth permittant for non-ruminants, the ionophores could eventually dominate the entire feed additive market.

Anthelmintic Agents. One antibiotic has been used as an anthelmintic agent for many years. Hygromycin B was isolated at the Lilly laboratories because of its antibacterial activity. Although it is active against both gram-positive and gram-negative bacteria, its activity was too weak to be therapeutically useful. It was tested in a variety of other assays and was found to be active in vivo against the pinworms, Aspicularis tetraptera and Syphacia obvelata. The anthelmintic activity was confirmed in pigs (12). It is licensed for the control of Ascaris galli, Heterakis gallinae and Capillaria obsignata in chickens when fed at the level of 8 to 12 g/ton an for the control of Ascaris suum, Oesophagostomum dentatum and Trichuris suis in swine, where it is fed at 12 g/ton.

A number of other fermentation products have been reported to have anthelmintic activity. Among these are the aminoglycoside, G-418, the destomycins, paromomycin, anthelvencin, aspiculamycin, anthelmycin, and the axenomycins. However, none of these has seen commercial use.

The third milestone in the history of the use of fermentation products in agriculture was the discovery of the avermectins. They were first detected in an anthelmintic assay using mice infected with nematospiroides dubius (13). This is one of the few assays in which they could have been detected since they lack antibacterial and antifungal activity.

Further experience has demonstrated that it was not solely the choice of assay but the great good fortune to have received a group of cultures from the Kitasato Institute and to have made the decision to screen these cultures in the N. dubius assay. One of these cultures, OS-3153, was active. The screening of several tens of thousands of soil isolates in this assay has failed to detect any remotely similar anthelmintic activity. Of the fermentation products discussed, this is the only one where the activity for which the product was eventually marketed was found by direct screening. (Zeranol might be considered to be another example, but it was not discovered by screening.)

Tests using helminth infections in a variety of laboratory animals soon revealed that the avermectins had activity against a variety of nematodes but lacked activity toward cestodes and trematodes. During the course of testing in a number of other assays, they were found active against the flour beetle, Tribolium confusum (14). This activity against arthropods was confirmed in mice infected with larvae of the bot fly, Cuterebra fontinella.

The avermectins are active against a wide variety of insects and other arthropods, including mites, ticks and lice. Moreover, they are active against nematode, insect and acarine infections of animals when administered in a single dose given orally or parenterally. Equally as exciting as their spectrum is their extreme potency. For example, avermectin B_{1a} exhibits greater than 95% efficacy against Haemonchus contortus, Ostertagia circumcincta, Trichostrongylus axei, T. colubriformis, Cooperia oncophora and Oesophagostomum columbianum when administered to sheep in a single oral dose of 100 µg/kg (15). It is even more potent against Ancylostoma caninum in dogs, where it is 83 to 100% effective when given as a single oral dose of 3 to 5 µg/kg (15). Undoubtedly the most sensitive ectoparasite is the larva of the common cattle grub, Hypoderma lineatum, where a single subcutaneous injection of 0.2 µg/kg gives 100% control (16).

This dual activity against both nematode and arthropod parasites of animals was an unexpected bonus from a screen for anthelmintic agents. The reason for this broad activity lies in their mode of action. They act by interfering with γ-aminobutyric acid (GABA) mediated neurotransmission. When treated with avermectin, the nematode Ascaris suum becomes paralyzed although it retains normal muscle tone (17). Picrotoxin, an antagonist of GABA, can reverse the effect of avermectin on neurotransmission in vitro. The absence of GABA-mediated neurotransmission in cestodes and trema-todes explains the lack of activity of the avermectins against these organisms.

The compound ultimately chosen for development was a semisynthetic derivative of the B_1 series in which the 22,23 double bond is reduced (18). The mixture consisting of at least 80% 22,23-dihydroavermectin B_{1a} and not more than 20% 22,23-dihydroavermectin B_{1b} has been named ivermectin. Its use level is 200 µg/kg in horses, cattle and sheep and 300 µg/kg in swine. It is injected subcutaneously in cattle and swine, and there are oral formulations for use in horses and sheep.

Plant Diseases

Fermentation products have played a rather minor role in the control of plant diseases. Table VI gives a classification of agents used on plants. These are divided into pesticides and growth modulators. The pesticides are classified as bactericides, fungicides, insecticides, miticides, nematicides and herbicides. There are fermentation products in each of these categories, and these are listed in Table VII.

Table VI. Classification of Agents Used on Plants

A. Pesticides
  1. Bactericides
  2. Fungicides
  3. Herbicides
  4. Insecticides
  5. Miticides
  6. Nematicides
B. Growth Modulators

It should be emphasized that although the total worldwide market for agricultural pesticides is huge (over $10 billion), the share held by fermentation products is quite small. Most of the fungicides listed in Table VII. are used in Japan, often for riceblast. There are several reasons for this small market share, but the most significant reason is probably economic. Although the fermentation products that have found commercial application are often much more active than chemical pesticides, this factor is not often sufficient to compensate for the higher cost of producing them.

Table VII. Fermentation Products Used on Plants

Name	Activity	Type	Used on:
Abamectin	Insecticide, miticide	Macrolide	Ornamentals
Aureofungin	Fungicide	Polyene	Fruits, vegetables(?)
Bialaphos	Herbicide	Phosphin. pept.	
Blasticidin S	Fungicide	Pyr. nucleoside	Rice
Cycloheximide	Fungicide, abscission agent	Glutarimide	Ornamentals, grass Citrus fruits, olives
Gibberelic Acid	Growth modulator	Diterpenoid	Fruits, vegetables
Kasugamycin	Fungicide	Aminocyclitol	Rice
Oxytetracycline	Bactericide, mycoplasmicide	Tetracycline	Fruits Palm trees
Pimaricin	Fungicide	Polyene	Bulbs
Polyoxin	Fungicide	Pyr. nucleoside	Rice, fruits, vegetables
Streptomycin	Bactericide	Aminocyclitol	Fruits, vegetables
Tetranactin	Miticide	Macrotetrolide	Fruits
Validamycin A	Fungistat	Aminocyclitol	Rice

There are a few companies that are hoping to change this. Several chemical companies that already have a large share of the chemical pesticide market are actively screening fermentation broths. A major motivation for this probably comes from the present concern about our environment. There is a perception that "natural" pesticides will have a much less serious environmental impact than "chemicals". Whether this advantage is real or only psychological remains to be seen.

Another incentive to this screening may have arisen from the discovery of two remarkably potent families of fermentation products with insecticidal and acaricidal activity, the milbemycins and the avermectins. Abamectin (a mixture of not less than 80% avermectin B_{1a} and not more than 20% avermectin B_{1b}) is already seeing limited use in Florida for the protection of ornamentals, and there is a considerable effort being made to develop the avermectins for use against a wide variety of insect and mite pests.

Two examples of the remarkable potency of avermectin B_{1a} are its LD_{90} of 0.02 to 0.03 ppm against the two-spotted spider mite, Tetranychus urticae, when applied to bean plants as a foliar spray; and its control of the red imported fire ant, Solenopsis invicta, when applied as a bait at a level as low as 25 to 50 mg per acre (19).

To express this extreme potency in another way, the spray for mites contains 4.5 mg of abamectin per liter whereas malathion spray, also used as a miticide, contains 3,700 mg per liter. This is over 800 times as much compound to produce the same effect.

Conclusion

Microorganisms are extremely versatile chemists. The wide variety of structures among the relatively few compounds discussed here is testimony to that. There are several theories to explain the evolutionary advantage conferred by the synthesis of secondary metabolites. (It often seems that they serve primarily to enrich pharmaceutical companies.) Until recently, the idea that they conferred a competitive advantage upon the producing organism seemed reasonable, since most of the products that had been detected had antibiotic activity.

For many years, screening programs were directed toward the discovery of antibacterial and antifungal antibiotics. Now the screening of microorganisms has shifted toward the search for other types of activities. Perhaps the products that had been found are more the result of the assays employed than of their synthetic capabilities. The ability to discover new types of fermentation products may be limited only by the ingenuity in developing new and sensitive assays along with a certain luck in selecting the proper microorganisms to test. The future for the use of fermentation products in agriculture holds much promise.

Acknowledgment

I wish to thank Dr. Robert Hamill of Lilly Research Laboratories for providing unpublished information about the discovery and development of monensin.

Literature Cited

1. Stokstad, E. L. R.; Jukes, T. H.; Pierce, J.; Page, A. C., Jr.; Franklin, A. L. J. Biol. Chem. 1949, 180, 647-654.
2. Ott, W. H.; Rickes, E. L.; Wood, T. L. J. Biol. Chem. 1948, 174, 1047-1048.
3. Stokstad, E. L. R.; Jukes, T. H. Proc. Soc. Exptl. Biol. Med. 1950, 73, 523-528.
4. Council for Agricultural Science and Technology. Report No. 88, Ames, Iowa 1981.
5. Hidy, P. H.; Baldwin, R. S.; Greasham, R. L.; Keith, C. L.; McMullen, J. R. Adv. Appl. Microbiol. 1977, 22, 59-82.
6. U. S. Office of Technology Assessment. "Drugs in Livestock Feed", Vol. I, Technical Report, U. S. Government Printing Office, Washington, D.C. 1979, 37.
7. Shumard, R. F; Callender, M. E. In: Hobby, G. L. (Ed.) Antimicrobial Agents and Chemotherapy - 1967, American Society for Microbiology, Ann Arbor, Mich. 1968, 369-377.
8. Berger, J.; Rachlin; A. I.; Scott, W. E.; Sternbach, L. H; Goldberg, M. W. J. Am. Chem. Soc. 1951, 73, 5295-5298.
9. Richardson, L. F.; Raun, A P.; Potter, E. L.; Cooley, C. O.; Rathmacher, R. P. J. Anim. Sci. 1974, 39, 250.
10. Leeson, S.; Hacker, R. H.; Wey, D. Can. J. Anim. Sci. 1981, 61, 1063-1065.
11. de Wilde, R. O. Deutsche Tierarztl. Wochenschr. 1984, 91, 22-24.
12. Goldsby, A. I.; Todd, A. C. North Amer. Vet. 1957, 38, 140-144.
13. Burg, R. W.; Miller, B. M; Baker, E. E.; Birnbaum, J.; Currie, S. A.; Hartman, R.; Kong, Y-L.; Monaghan, R. L.; Olson, G.; Putter, I.; Tunac, J. B.; Wallick, H.; Stapley, E. O.; Oiwa, R; Omura, S. Antimicrob. Agents Chemother. 1979, 15, 361-367.
14. Ostlind, D. A.; Cifelli, S; Long, R. Vet. Rec. 1979, 105, 168.
15. Egerton, J. R.; Ostlind, D. A.; Blair, L. S.; Eary, C. H.; Suhayda, D.; Cifelli, S.; Riek, R. F; Campbell, W. C. Antimicrob. Agents Chemother. 1979, 15, 372-378.
16. Drummond, R. O. J. Econ. Entomol 1984,, 77, 402-406.
17. Kass, I. W.; Wang, C. C.; Walrond, J. P; Stretton, A. O. W. Proc. Nat. Acad. Sci. U.S. 1980, 77, 6211-6215.
18. Chabala, J. C.; Mrozik, H; Tolman, R. L.; Eskola, P.; Lusi, A.; Peterson, L. H.; Woods, M. F.; Fisher, M. H.; Campbell, W. C.; Egerton, J. R.; Ostlind, D. A. J. Med. Chem. 1980, 23, 1134-1136.
19. Campbell, W. C.; Burg, R. W.; Fisher, M. H; Dybas, R. A. in Magee, P. S.; Kohn, G. K; Menn, J. J. (Eds.) Pesticide Synthesis Through Rational Approaches, A.C.S. Symposium Series 255, American Chemical Society, Washington, D.C. 1984, 5-20.
20. Aronson, C. E. (Ed.) Veterinary Pharmaeuticals & Biologicals 1982/1983, Veterinary Medicine Publishing Co., Edwardsville, Kansas, 1983.
21. Leidahl, R. (Ed.) 1985 Feed Additive Compendium, The Miller Publishing Company, Minneapolis, Minnesota, 1984.

RECEIVED February 18, 1986

RISKS AND BENEFITS

7

Benefits and Risks of Antibiotics Use in Agriculture

Virgil W. Hays

Department of Animal Sciences, University of Kentucky, Lexington, KY 40546-0215

The advisability of using certain antibiotics, particularly penicillin and tetracycline, in animal feeds has been questioned because of their use in human medicine. Any use of an antibiotic that is prescribed for humans presents some risks to human health, whether the use is for humans, animals or for other purposes; but, the uses also have benefits. Otherwise, they would not persist. Antibiotics are used in animal feeds to increase animal weight, increase efficiency of feed utilization, increase reproductive efficiency and decrease morbidity and mortality. These benefits to animals and animal producers are reflected in decreases in food costs to humans. There are also benefits to human health from use of antibiotics in food animals. By reducing the incidence of animal health problems, use of antibiotics in food animals reduce the transference of animal infections to humans. The contention that the effectiveness of penicillin and tetracycline for use in human medicine is rapidly diminishing as a result of the proliferation of resistant bacteria caused by subtherapeutic use of antibiotics in animal production is not supported by experimental data. Rather, the evidence suggests that a fairly stable level of resistance of the intestinal bacteria in humans has long since been established to penicillin and tetracycline as it has been in animals.

For the past 35 years, U.S. livestock and poultry producers have used antibiotics (products of microbial synthesis) and chemotherapeutics (chemically synthesized products). The drugs are administered in relatively large dosages to treat sick animals (therapeutically) and in lower dosages to prevent disease in exposed animals (prophylactically). More commonly, small amounts (subtherapeutic) of antibiotics are added to animal feeds to prevent or reduce diseases and to improve feed efficiency and growth.

Approximately 80% of the poultry, 75% of the swine, 60% of the beef cattle and 75% of the dairy calves marketed are estimated to have received antibiotics at some time in their life (CAST, 3). Of the antibiotics produced each year in the U.S., 45 to 55% are administered to animals.

Three broad groupings, of the antibiotic substances presently used in animal production, include: (a) broad-spectrum antibiotics, including penicillins and tetracyclines, which are effective against a wide variety of pathogenic and non-pathogenic bacteria; (b) several narrow-spectrum antibiotics that are not used in human medicine; and, (c) the ionophore antibiotics, monensin, lasalocid and salinomycin. Monensin and lasalocid are used as rumen fermentation regulators in beef cattle, and the three ionophores are used as coccidiostats in poultry production. The ionophores, which are not used in human medicine, were first introduced in the 1970's and account for most of the increase in antibiotic usage in animal production since the 1960's.

Why Are Antibiotics Used In Animal Production?

The efficacy of antibiotics in improving rate and efficiency of growth has been well documented by many researchers. To illustrate the responses in animals, a comprehensive summary involving 937 experiments and more than 20,000 pigs is presented in table 1. Note

Table 1. Response of Pigs to Subtherapeutic Levels of Antibiotics[1]

Item	Control	Antibiotic	Improvement, %
Starter phase (15-57 lb)			
Average daily gain, lb	.86	1.01	16
Feed/gain	2.32	2.16	7
Grower phase (37-108 lb)			
Average daily gain, lb	1.30	1.45	11
Feed/gain	2.91	2.78	5
Grower-finisher phase (44-189 lb)			
Average daily gain, lb	1.50	1.56	4
Feed/gain	3.37	3.30	2

[1] Data from 378, 280 and 279 experiments, involving 10,023, 4,783 and 5,666 pigs for the three phases, respectively (Hays, 5).

that the magnitude of the response is greater for the younger animals and declines as the animal matures. Similar results could be presented for chicks, turkeys and cattle. For the most part, the summary presented is based on data from Experiment Station or Industry research units. We have relatively few published experiments carried out in a production environment. Such overall summaries as the one in table 1 markedly underestimate the total benefits derived from antibiotics for three major reasons: (1) the data for the more as well as the less effective antibiotics are pooled; (2) growth rate and feed conversion are accounted for, but reduction in mortality and improved reproductive performance are not appropriately considered; and, (3) the magnitude of the responses is smaller in the experiment station environment than in commercial production unit environments. This latter effect on estimates of the average benefits is illustrated by the data presented in table 2. By pooling a large number of observations as was done for this table, to overcome at least partially the biological variation

Table 2. Comparison of Response to Antibacterial Agents by Pigs in Experiment Station and Production Unit Environments [1]

Location	No. Experiments	% Improvement from Antibiotics [2]	
		Daily gain	Feed/gain
Experiment station research units	128	16.9	7.0
Production units	32	28.4	14.5
Weight avg.	160	19.2	8.5

[1] Data on 12,000 pigs from 15 to 57 lb. (Hays, 5).

[2] Chlortetracycline-penicillin-sulfamethazine, tylosin-sulfamethazine, tetracyclines and carbadox.

associated with small experiments, one can illustrate that the responses to antibiotics by young pigs in production units are nearly twice that observed in Experiment Station units.

There are several reasons why the Experiment Station or Industry research unit data are likely to underestimate the real benefits from antibiotics. These include: (1) Animals are selected for uniformity, and any poor-doing or unhealthy animals are not used unless the experiment is specifically designed for that purpose. The producer must treat if necessary, allow the unhealthy animals to recover, and, to the extent practical, finish all animals. Ample data are available to illustrate that the response to antibiotics is much greater in poorly-doing animals. (2) The environment of the animals is less conducive to stress conditions in most experimental situations than may be practical for commercial operations. Animals are grouped in smaller numbers and frequently the space allowance is excessive. (3) Sanitation is usually better in the experimental situation, particularly for pigs and poultry, in that buildings are usually emptied, cleaned and disinfected between experiments. (4) Ration-balancing and feeding procedures are generally more precise and ingredient quality is closely monitored in most experimental situations.

Some critics of current commercial production methods suggest that antibiotics are necessary only because of the stressful rearing conditions and that the return to more extensive rearing systems would obviate the need for antibiotics. Returning to the extensive animal rearing systems would result in exposure to greater environmental extremes and increase the exposure to internal parasites and the associated susceptibility to diseases, hence would increase rather than decrease the response to antibacterial agents.

Improved performance of the animals and reduced mortality are definite benefits. The total aggregate of these benefits to all of animal agriculture is very substantial and has been estimated to be as much as a $3.5 billion per year reduction in food costs to the U.S. consuming public (CAST, 3).

Why the Concern About Using Antibiotics In Animal Production?

Since 1977, the Food and Drug Adminstration (FDA) has been considering a ban on the subtherapeutic use of procaine penicillin and tetracyclines in animal feeds. These antibiotics are used in both humans and animals, and any use of an antibiotic that is prescribed for humans presents some risk to human health, whether the use is for humans, animals, or other purposes. The risk is that pathogenic or disease-causing bacteria may develop a strain that resists that antibiotic. The resistant strain of the pathogen then may cause human disease that cannot be treated by this antibiotic.

The risk that exists from the use of antibiotics in animals arises through a complicated series of events. When an antibiotic is fed to an animal, it comes in contact with the vast and complex bacterial population in the digestive tract. If present in biologically effective amounts, it affects the sensitive bacteria, which may include pathogens; but, the total number of living bacteria remains about the same. The sensitive bacteria destroyed or inhibited, and the resistant bacteria multiply to take their place. These resistant bacteria may contaminate animal products used by humans as food.

Two types of bacterial resistance to antibiotics are known: (a) resistance due to genes transferred to the progeny via the chromosome--the regular, relatively stable genetic material and (b) resistance due to transfer of genes on "R plasmids", which are bits of genetic material smaller than chromosomes that exist and replicate autonomously in the cell cytoplasm. The transfer of resistance due R plasmids is not necessarily limited to other bacteria of the same genus or species, and R plasmids may also carry other genetic factors that increase or decrease the virulence of the organisms to which they are transferred (Fagerberg et al., 4). Another problem results from the fact that resistance to one antibiotic may be genetically linked in some instances to resistance to one or more other antibiotics.

Both types of resistance in animal bacteria can affect human health. Bacteria of animal origin that are resistant to a particular antibiotic may make this antibiotic ineffective for controlling human infections with pathogens bearing the kind of resistance carried by these bacteria as a consequence of (a) the pathogenic properties of the animal bacteria as such, or (b) the transference of the resistance to other bacteria, which may be human pathogens. The transfer may occur in either animals or humans, and if conditions are right for bacterial growth, the transfer could take place in a prepared food.

Are Antibiotic Residues A Concern?

Another frequently cited concern to humans from use of antibiotics in animal feeds is that the residues in the edible animal products may increase the human intake of antibiotics, and thus cause development of antibiotic-resistant pathogenic bacteria in humans. To avoid this possibility, FDA establishes maximum levels that can be used in animal feeds and a minimum time interval between the last use of feed containing antibiotics and the slaughter of the animals. This allows for elimination of antibiotics from the animals before slaughter. A review of the U.S. Department of Agriculture's monitoring records confirms that antibiotic residues in animal products are not a significant problem. If antibiotics did remain in the tissues, they would be inactivated by cooking.

Certain of the chemotherapeutics, for example the sulfa drugs, have been of greater concern from the point of view of tissue residues. Though there is no evidence that the sulfa residues found in pork livers or kidneys has or would cause human health problems, they are violative by our present standards. Therapeutic use (high dosages) of antibiotics are more likely to result in residues than are feed additive uses, but it is important that only approved levels and required withdrawal periods be adhered to for all drugs.

Is Subtherapeutic Antibiotic Use A Contributor To Human Health Problems?

The current concern about subtherapeutic doses of antibiotics in animal feeds gained renewed impetus from two scientific papers (Holmberg et al., 7-8), by researchers at the Centers for Disease Control (CDC) in Atlanta and a related editorial (Levy, 11) and news articles (Sun, 16-7) in scientific journals about them.

In early 1983, Dr. Scott Holmberg (a CDC epidemiologist) and his colleagues identified 18 persons in four midwestern states who were affected by a severe diarrhea caused by a strain of Salmonella newport that was resistant to tetracycline, as well as ampicillin and carbenicillin (chemically synthesized relatives of penicillin). Of these 18 persons, 13 had consumed hamburger supplied directly from a particular herd of cattle, or they had purchased hamburger from markets thought to be supplied with meat from the herd. The cattle in question were produced in a feedlot in South Dakota, where they had received feed containing chlortetracycline at a subtherapeutic level.

Some supporters of the proposed FDA ban on the use of subtherapeutic levels of penicillin and tetracyclines in animal feeds hailed the results of the CDC study as a clear link between subtherapeutic antibiotic use in food animal production and antibiotic-resistant diseases in humans. Some opponents, on the other hand, pointed to the lack of evidence needed to constitute adequate scientific proof that the resistant organism came from hamburger, that the hamburger was contaminated with the resistant strain of <u>Salmonella newport</u>, that if the hamburger was contaminated, the source of contamination was the herd of cattle implicated, that the herd itself harbored the resistant organism, or that subtherapeutic usage of chlortetracycline had any connection to the antibiotic resistance of the organism or its proliferation.

The really important point is not whether this particular CDC investigation did or did not demonstrate the link, but rather, are there problems; and, if so, how important are the problems resulting from use of antibiotics at subtherapeutic levels in animal feeds? In other words, would discontinuing the subtherapeutic use of tetracycline and penicillin have a significant effect on antibiotic resistance in consumers of animal products?

Long Term Experiments On Impact of Antibiotic Restrictions

In addition to our work on the animal responses to antibiotics, we have been very much involved in the impact of antibacterial agents on the microflora of the animals and their environment. Since 1972 we have monitored the level and patterns of resistance in two separate herds of pigs and have used pigs from these herds in experiments conducted at a third location. In the control herd, we have used antibiotics much as a swine producer would except that a portion of the herd has been continuously exposed to tetracycline antibiotics at a level of 50 to 100 grams per ton of feed. The other herd, a Specific Pathogen Free herd located at our Princeton, Kentucky Experiment Station, has had no exposure to any antibacterial agent for therapeutic or subtherapeutic purposes since the project was started (May, 1972). This herd (antibiotic-free herd) is completely isolated from other pigs. Any new genetic material is introduced into the herd by artificial insemination of selected females to provide the required number of males. All diets have been prepared on the research farm and no antibiotic containing feeds have been processed in that mill. No animal products are included in the diet in order to limit diet as an entry source for resistant organisms.

These two herds have provided information on development, persistency and transfer of antibacterial resistance; and, furthermore, they have provided information regarding the impact the previously proposed restrictions (Fed. Reg. 42:43770 and 42:52645, 1977) of antibiotic usage would have on antibiotic resistant bacteria of animal origin as a health hazard to humans.

Following antibiotic withdrawal, the performance of pigs in the antibiotic-free herd was markedly reduced (Langlois et al., <u>9-10</u>). Conception rate on first service declined (91% vs. 84%), sows farrowed fewer pigs (10.9 vs. 10.1), fewer pigs survived to weaning (8.9 vs. 7.5), and the pigs were smaller at three-week weaning (12.1 lb. vs. 11.5 lb.). We realize that such before- and after-withdrawal comparisons alone are not valid estimates of the average benefits of feed additive usage of antibiotics. However, the differences observed are remarkably similar to the average responses from controlled experiments.

Numerous other problems have been encountered since antibiotics were discontinued. A higher proportion of the pigs do poorly (runt pigs) resulting in more variable as well as an overall increase in length of time to reach market weight. There has been an increase in the incidence of mastitis, metritis and agalactia, 10% (before) vs. 66% (after) of sows affected. There has been a greater incidence of lameness and skeletal joint problems. On several occasions, the pigs have had severe skin lesions attributed to staphylococcal infections. Two recent outbreaks of diarrhea were diagnosed as porcine proliferated enteritis with <u>Campylobacter</u> diagnosed as the causative organism. Conversely, we have not encountered similar or other major health problems in the control (continuous-antibiotic) herd.

Antibiotic Use and Bacterial Resistance

It may conceivably be argued that no one has proposed a complete ban on antibiotic usage, and that these studies would not be useful in evaluating the effects of restricted antibiotic use. However, the impact any restrictions would have on antibiotic resistance must be considered in evaluating the effectiveness of alternatives other than a complete ban. We have monitored the level and pattern of antibiotic resistance in enteric bacteria at periodic intervals during the past 13 years. Initially, the enteric bacteria of the two herds did not differ greatly in level or pattern of resistance. Though there had been no specifically planned use of antibiotics in these research herds and no one antibiotic had been used continuously at either location, antibiotics were used experimentally or as a swine producer would use them.

As one would expect, after 13 years of continuous exposure, the levels of antibiotic resistance and levels of multiple resistance are higher in the control herd. In that herd, tetracycline resistance in the fecal coliform populations has remained high, averaging more than 90%. Tetracycline resistance of the fecal coliforms in the antibiotic-free herd has declined from the initial high level of above 90%; but, the resistance level still fluctuates between 20 and 55% even though these animals have had no exposure to antibiotics for 13 years. During that time more than 5 complete generation turn-overs of that herd have occurred. We have monitored the resistance to 14 antimicrobial agents; and, the fecal coliforms, on the average, are resistant to 1.5 to 2.0 of those agents (table 3).

Factors Affecting Resistance to Antibiotics

We find that the level of antibiotic resistance is related to or influenced by a number of factors including age of animal, with organisms from younger pigs having a higher level of resistance than that of more mature animals. After 11 years of no antibiotic exposure, approximately 55% of the fecal coliforms from pigs less than six months of age were resistant to tetracycline; and, on the average were resistant to 2.9 of the 14 agents tested. In more mature pigs (6 months or older) the level of tetracycline resistance was about 25%; and, on the average, the fecal coliforms were resistant to about 1.5 agents.

Table 3. Tetracycline Resistance in Fecal Coliforms of Pigs in Antibiotic-free Herd (No Antibiotics Since 1972)

Age of pig, months	No. isolates	Tetracycline resistance %	Multiple resistance[1] no.
All isolates (1972-1982)			
2-6	977	73	2.5
7-11	358	26	1.1
12-23	701	35	1.5
23	370	30	1.5
Samples, March '83			
2-6	161	55	2.9
7-11	51	24	1.6
12-23	47	26	1.4
23	21	24	1.7

[1] Average number of antibacterials to which fecal coliforms were resistant.

We have found that stressing pigs by transporting them to another location will increase the level of resistance and will also increase shedding of lactose-negative coliforms (including Salmonella). These effects are very obvious when the travel is quite distant; but, similar, though smaller in magnitude, effects are noted when animals are transported less than 10 miles. For example, pigs were sampled prior to and after being transported 200 miles. The level of tetracycline resistance increased from 40% to a level of 80% as a result of the stress of moving. Several days were required for the levels of resistance to return to the previously lower level. We have also noted that stressing pigs by forcing them to walk for about 0.5 miles will increase the percentage of fecal coliforms resistant to tetracyclines.

Short Term Therapeutic Use and Bacterial Resistance

Exposure of animals to therapeutic levels of antibiotics will markedly raise the level of resistance, and a long period of time is required for the resistance levels to return to the pre-treatment level. In an experiment replicated five times (Langlois et al. 10), we found that exposure of animals to subtherapeutic levels of gram-positive spectrum antibiotics also resulted in increased levels of tetracycline resistance. During the course of our study we have sampled pigs on two separate occasions (1974 and 1985) from another research herd in which antibiotics have never been used as feed additives, but only for therapeutic purposes. Of the 100 pigs sampled in 1974, only one had been treated and that pig was treated more than a year prior to sampling. Antibiotic resistance levels in that herd were between our two herds with 72% of the fecal coliforms in the first sampling being resistant (by the disc plate technique) to tetracycline (Hays and Muir, 6). In 1985, 76% of the fecal coliforms were resistant (using the Sensititre MIC/ID System, 8 mcg/ml).

The results from our studies make it very clear that the previous proposal [Fed. Reg. 42:43770 (Aug. 30, 1977) and Fed. Reg. 42:52645 (Oct. 21, 1977), as endorsed in the petition from the Natural Resources Defense Council (NRDC, Fed. Reg. 49:49645, December 21, 1984)] for restricting feed additive use of subtherapeutic levels of penicillin and tetracycline, would have very little, if any, impact on the levels or patterns of antibiotic resistance in food-producing animals and the resulting exposure of humans to resistant bacteria of animal origin.

For livestock producers to approach the care we have exercised in in avoiding antibiotic exposure would require a complete ban of all antibiotics and other antibacterial agents. Periodic exposure to prophylactic or therapeutic levels of antibacterials would result in high levels of resistance and, in a production environment, that resistance would be very slow in declining.

Human Health Implications

The results of the Seattle-King County (Nolan et al. 12) study are very supportive of the conclusions we have drawn from our experiments. Incidence of **Salmonella** and **Campylobacter** contamination and antibiotic resistance levels of these bacteria associated with processing plants and retail meats were as high or higher in poultry products than for other meats. Of the strains isolated from retail poultry, 33% of the **Campylobacter jejuni** strains and 31% of the **Salmonella** strains showed resistance to tetracyclines. Since the introduction of the ionophore antibiotics to control coccidiosis (1971), there has been little, if any, subtherapeutic use of tetracyclines or penicillin in broiler production. Furthermore, broiler production and processing and the manufacturing of broiler feeds are largely separated from any aspect of swine and beef production and processing. Thus, in essence, we have experienced a 15 year, large scale test on the impact of the proposed actions and found it to be nil.

In 1971, Great Britain implemented a ban on subtherapeutic use of tetracyclines in animal production. This action was taken after considerable debate and was greatly influenced by antibiotic resistant **Salmonella** infections (**S. typhimurium** phage type 29) in humans in the mid-1960's, which appeared to be related to similar infections in calves (Anderson, 2). Antibiotics were not approved as feed additives for calves at that time nor previously. Thus, earlier implementation of the Swann Committee (18) recommendations would have had no apparent impact on that particular epidemic, nor did it prevent a similar epidemic later (Rowe et al., 13).

Dr. B. Rowe, Director of the Central Public Health Laboratory, London, participated in the July 19-20, 1984 International Symposium on **Salmonella**, in New Orleans. He was quoted in Food Chemical News (Aug. 6, 1984, page 17) as follows: "the British increase in cases of salmonellosis caused by multiple-drug-resistant forms of **S.**

typhimurium is totally due to injudicious use of antibiotics in animal husbandry". If one accepted this sweeping but unsubstantiated conclusion, then one would logically conclude that the prohibition of subtherapeutic use in animals of those antibiotics used in human medicine has had no impact on the situation in Great Britain.

Smith (14) reported a slight decrease in tetracycline-resistant Escherichia coli, but the number of pigs excreting these organisms did not change during the 4-year period after implementation of the Swann Report recommendations by the British Government. Some have attributed a lack of change in resistance levels among the organisms from animals in Great Britain to injudicious use of antibiotics through producers and veterinarians finding ways to circumvent the regulations. Our research would indicate that on discontinuing subtherapeutic use of antibiotics, incidence of disease problems would increase, thus necessitating an increased need for therapeutic use. Furthermore, periodic therapeutic use would result in continued excretion of antibiotic resistant organisms. Though our research experiences are supportive of a lack of impact on antibiotic resistance in Great Britain from the withdrawal of subtherapeutic use in animals, we certainly could not agree with the statement attributed to Rowe that multi-drug-resistant Salmonella in humans is totally due to drug use in animals as Rowe concluded.

The recent report (Holmberg et al., 7) on the Salmonella newport epidemic in Minnesota and South Dakota has been highly publicized and proclaimed as the "direct link" or "smoking gun" that ties feed additive use of tetracyclines in beef cattle to serious human health problems. Much speculation was required to link the infective Salmonella to that particular beef farm and even further to conclude that subtherapeutic use of antibiotics in the cattle either resulted in the development of the resistance pattern or resulted in selecting for the organism. The authors correctly acknowledged that the organism was not found on that beef farm nor in ground beef. They further acknowledged that the resistance pattern (tetracycline-ampicillin-carbenicillin) of the S. newport organism most likely did not develop on that farm. However, the thesis presented to the public by the media is as follows: the organism entered that group of beef cattle by some means, possibly a stray calf from a neighboring farm, and the use of a tetracycline gave the Salmonella organism the selective advantage for rapid proliferation. In reality, if tetracycline was used with any regularity on that farm, the tetracycline resistant Salmonella would have had little, if any, selective advantage because of its tetracycline resistance, as the majority of the resident gram-negative organisms would have been resistant to tetracycline.

No factual evidence was presented to demonstrate that the resistant Salmonella newport organism did gain entrance to that beef herd. If, however, the organism did enter the herd, a selective advantage could have been provided equally as or more likely by the use of a gram-positive spectrum antibacterial agent, a change in the diet of the animals, a disruption of feed intake triggered by inclement weather, or the stress of transporting those animals to these are mere speculations; but, we have research data to support each of them as factors capable of triggering the proliferation of a previously asymptomatic infection.

The authors (Holmberg et al. 7) did not rule out sources other than that beef herd, for the S. newport bacteria. If one assumes that infected hamburger did come through that brokerage firm and from that Nebraska processor, the total carcass weight from 59 cattle probably would not be as much as 41,000 lbs. (62% yield on 1100 lb. cattle). Considerably less than that would have gone into boxed beef and/or hamburger. There was probably no more than 29,000 pounds after fat, bone and waste trim and only about 7000 lb. of that, at the most, would be hamburger. Where did the other 41,000 to 63,000 lbs. (70,000-29,000 or 7000) come from? Why wasn't there any human illness that could be linked to the 46 cattle that went through other processors? Could it be that the original source of those 59 cattle had nothing to do with the illness incidents? Granted that all people infected with Salmonella do not become ill and/or are not identified; but, it seems highly unlikely that one can divide a group of infected cattle nearly in half and send one half through one chain and result in 12 identified cases of illness and the other half through another route and result in no identifiable cases. Wouldn't it be equally or more likely that the Salmonella originated in the beef that was mixed with that of the 59 carcasses? Furthermore, the authors did not demonstrate that subtherapeutic use of tetracycline was related in any way to the illness of the patients. If one makes a third assumption that the infective Salmonella did originate in the hamburger from those 59 carcasses from that South Dakota Farm, the use of antibiotics could have been unrelated to the chain of events. The Salmonella newport strain isolated from ill patients and a dairy calf that died on a farm adjacent to the beef farm was resistant to tetracycline, ampicillin and carbenicillin. Ampicillin and carbenicillin are not used in beef cattle except possibly on a prescription basis and not likely then. The authors did not report illness in the beef animals and further they state: "Thus, the beef herd was probably not the original source of the R plasmid, but the use of subtherapeutic tetracycline in the herd's feed throughout 1982 provided a selective pressure for persistence of the antimicrobial resistant organism".

One can readily see that the conclusions of the authors are based on numerous assumptions rather than on factual data. Unfortunately, this is the nature of retrospective epidemiological studies. One cannot really fault the authors for their sequence of theories leading them to a possible source of the infections. Such efforts are necessary for sorting out the potential source of infections; and, through follow-up studies and designed experiments, we can determine sources of infections and methods for prevention. They evidently did omit some observations on the meat samples they did check and observations on the adjacent dairy herd; and, they did not take samples from the cattle's environment on the beef farm. If the beef farm was thought to be the source, there should have been more effort to find the organism on that farm.

Antibiotic Resistance and Virulence

The Natural Resources Defense Council petition infers from calculations based on a very small number of observations that antibiotic resistant Salmonella are more virulent, hence result in more deaths than do antibiotic-sensitive Salmonella (Ahmed et al., 1). Controlled experiments with chicks on the effects of the resistance carrying plasmids on virulence of Salmonella led Smith (15) to the following conclusion: "The mortality rates from infection with the R+ (resistant) strains were similar to, slightly lower than, or much lower than those from infections with corresponding R- (sensitive) strains". Numerous reports support Smith's conclusions.

In the more recent Chicago outbreak of Salmonellosis, which has been attributed to milk contaminated with a tetracycline-resistant strain of Salmonella typhimurium, there were two deaths verified as resulting from infections with the resistant strain of Salmonella in 16,284 confirmed cases. If one pools these cases with those cited in the NRDC petition, then the incidence of mortality (0.09%) is similar or than that of persons affected by antibiotic-sensitive Salmonella (0.21%) also cited by NRDC. Thus, the similarity of risks of human infections with resistant and sensitive strains of Salmonella agrees with research data obtained in controlled experiments (Smith 15).

Reducing Human Exposure

I do not wish to leave the impression that I'm unaware of the importance of bacterial contamination of animal products. There is no question about the significance of Salmonella and Campylobacter jejuni being a problem in human health, and food producing animals serve along with pets, humans, wildlife and other foods as a part of the total Salmonella- Campylobacter reservoir. There are very serious questions, however, regarding the impact of antibiotic usage in animals on antibiotic resistance in humans. There is a great deal of research evidence to indicate that the action proposed, to restrict certain uses of tetracyclines and penicillin, would have essentially no impact on human exposure to antibiotic resistant organisms. Implementing the proposed action would have an adverse impact on the production costs of animal products. We do need means for markedly reducing or completely eliminating bacterial contamination. An earlier CDC report (Holmberg et al., 1984b) indicates there are added risks associated with consumption of raw meats and milk. Thus, using pasteurized milk only and proper handling and cooking of meats are important precautions for preventing food borne illnesses. Other useful means for reducing the health risks from bacterial contaminants of animal products and other foods include public education on personal hygiene of all food handlers and appropriate cooking and handling techniques for all foods.

Literature Cited

1. Ahmed, A. K., S. Chasis and B. McBarnette. "Petition of the Natural Resources Defense Council, Inc. to the Secretary of Health and Human Services requesting immediate suspension of approval of the subtherapeutic use of penicillin and tetracyclines in animal feeds"; Nov. 20. NRDC, New York, NY. 1984.

2. Anderson, E.S. "Observations on ecological effects of antibacterial drugs"; in Dunlop, R. H. and Moon, H. W., Eds.; Resistance to Infectious Disease, Saskatoon Modern Press, Saskatoon, Saskatchewan, 1970, pp 157-172.

3. CAST. "Antibiotics in Animal Feeds"; Council for Agricultural Science and Technology. Ames, IA. Rpt. No. 88, 1981.

4. Fagerberg, D. J., Quarles, C. L.; McKinley, G. A. Antibiotic resistance and its transfer; Feed Management June, 1979, pp 32, 34 and 37.

5. Hays, V. W. "Effectiveness of Feed Additive Usage of Antibacterial Agents in Swine and Poultry Production"; Rachelle Lab., Long Beach, CA. 1977.

6. Hays, V. W.; Muir, W. M. Efficacy and safety of feed additive use of antibacterial drugs in animal production. Can. J. Animal Sci., 1978, 59,447.

7. Holmberg, S. D.; Osterholm, M. T.; Senger, K. A.; Cohen, M. L. Drug resistant Salmonella from animals fed antimicrobials. New England Journal of Medicine, 1984, 311,617.

8. Holmberg, S. D.; Wells, J. G.; Cohen, M. L. Animal-to-man transmission of antimicrobial-resistant Salmonella: Investigations of U. S. Outbreaks, 1971-1983. Science 1984, 225,833.

9. Langlois, B. E.; Cromwell, G. L.; Hays, V. W. Influence of chlortetracycline in swine feed on reproductive performance and on incidence and persistence of antibiotic resistant enteric bacteria. J. Animal Sci., 1978, 46, 1369.

10. Langlois, B. E.; Cromwell, G. L.; Hays, V. W. Influence of type of antibiotic and length of antibiotic feeding period on performance and persistence of antibiotic resistant enteric bacteria in growing finishing swine. J. Animal Sci., 1978, 46, 1383.

11. Levy, S. B. Playing antibiotic pool: Time to tally the score. New England Journal of Medicine. 1984, 311, 663.

12. Nolan, C. M.; Harris, N. V.; Canova, P. M.; Skillman, S. M.; Cain-Nelson, A. K.; Tenover, F. C.; Coyle, M. B.; Plorde, J. J.; Weiss, N. S.; Martin, D. C. Surveillance of the Flow of Salmonella and Campylobacter in a Community. Prepared for the U. S. Department of Health and Human Services, Public Health Service, Food and Drug Administration, Bureau of Veterinary Medicine. Contract No. 223-81-7041. Communicable Disease Control Section, Seattle-King County (Washington) Department of Public Health. 1984.

13. Rowe, B.; Threlfall, E. J.; Ward, L. R.; Ashley, A. S. International spread of multiresistant strains of *Salmonella typhimurium* phage types 204 and 193 from Britain to Europe. Vet Record, 1979, 105, 468.

14. Smith, H. W. "Antibiotic resistant bacteria and associated problems before and after the 1969 Swann Report". in Woodbine, M. Ed. Antibiotics and Antibiosis in Agriculture. Butterworths, London. 1977.

15. Smith, H. W. The effect on virulence of transferring R factors to *Salmonella typhimurium in vivo*. J. Med. Microbiol. 1972, 5, 451.

16. Sun, M. In search of *Salmonella's* smoking gun. Science 1984, 226, 30.

17. Sun, M. Use of antibiotics in animal feed challenged. Science, 1984, 226, 144.

18. Swann, M. M. Report of Joint Committee on the Use of Antibiotics in Animal Husbandry and Veterinary Medicine. Cmnd. 4198, Her Majesty's Stationery Office, London. 1969.

RECEIVED May 5, 1986

8

Significance of Antibiotics in Foods and Feeds

Khem M. Shahani and Paul J. Whalen

Department of Food Science and Technology, University of Nebraska, Lincoln, NE 68583-0919

> The use of antibiotics in livestock production for increased feed efficiency is widespread. Such use may indirectly access human food in the form of residuals in products such as meat and milk. For years, scientists and health officials have warned of the risk of developing resistant pathogens from feeding antibiotics to livestock. Recently, this concern was fueled by a fatal case of salmonellosis caused by an antibiotic resistant strain linked to meat. Failure to withhold milk produced after treating mastitic or otherwise diseased animals is the primary cause of antibiotics in milk. Lactic cultures produce inherent antibiotics active against a wide range of pathogenic and nonpathogenic bacteria. The benefits of the naturally occurring antibiotics produced in fermented milk products are being investigated for use in treating E. coli mediated diarrhea and Salmonella/Shigella dysentery in children. Although the economic advantages of incorporating antibiotics in animal feed for livestock production are massive, the risk to the consumer must be weighed against such advantages.

The advent of antibiotics began a new era in the treatment of human and animal disease. Initially, antibiotics were used in a therapeutic mode only. However, in the early 1950 s, it was discovered that the residual mash from chlortetracycline production produced a growth promoting effect on chicks which was later attributed to low levels of the antibiotic present in the mash. Use of antibiotics in feeds for animal production has grown to account for about half of over 35 million lbs produced annually in the U.S. ([1](#)). Concern that this extensive use may be compromising human therapeutic use is mounting due to increasing prevalence of multiply antibiotic resistant intestinal bacteria, not only in the flora of the treated animal, but in the producer personnel as well. Of principal concern are the complications presented by pathogens such as salmonella whose DNA containing plasmids (R factor) allow acquisition of multiple resistance and present serious, potentially fatal, illness upon transmission to humans.

Antibiotics in Foods and Feeds

Antibiotic residuals in food products are considered additives by the FDA. Therefore, such products are considered adulterated and restricted from interstate commerce. In addition, widespread use of antibiotics for food production may pose the risk of toxic or allergic reactions in sensitized individuals. Cultures employed in fermented dairy products such as cheese or yogurt are extremely susceptible to low levels of antibiotics in the milk supply where production schedules may be thrown off and product losses incurred due to the presence of antibiotics. Alternatively, some lactic cultures synthesize natural antibacterial, antibiotic-like compounds active against a wide range of pathogenic and nonpathogenic bacteria. In view of some adverse effects of antibiotic feeding, use of these probiotics is being promoted. Several countries other than the U.S. permit the use of nisin in dairy products as a bacteriocin which is not therapeutically employed in man or animals.

Antibiotic resistant microorganisms. Livestock production employs antibiotics in 3 basic manners (2):
1) Therapeutic - treatment of disease and infection
2) Prophylaxis - disease prevention in healthy animals
3) Growth promotion - continual subtherapeutic or low doses of antibiotics in normal, healthy animals for improved production (growth rate and/or feed efficiency).

Therapeutic levels of antibiotics range from 200 - 500 g/ton while prophylactic applications range from 50 - 200 g/ton and subtherapeutic levels in feed range from 1 - 50 g/ton for poultry, swine and calves (3). It is the long term or continual incorporation of antibiotics in feeds which concerns many scientists in that many of the antibiotics used for production purposes are also used for therapy in man. As will be discussed, the resistant organisms which result from antibiotics in feeds can subvert, potentially, therpeutic application of these drugs should the resistant organisms present a pathogenic situation in man.

The presence of antibiotic resistant intestinal organisms resulting from the use of antibiotics in feeds is well established (4, 5, 6). Wanatabe (7) reported on the transferability of this trait and Anderson and Lewis (8) showed the transfer of antibiotic resistance between species involving Salmonella typhimurium. Siegel et al. (5) showed the effect of antibiotic feeds on the number of antibiotic resistant E. coli in swine, poultry and cattle as compared to range cattle. As shown in Table I, extremely high percentiles of resistant cultures were found in the animals on feed versus very low levels in the range cattle. The spread of these resistant fecal flora to man has been demonstrated by Levy et al. (6). In this study, the farm personnel acquired a significantly higher population of tetracycline resistant coliforms (mainly E. coli) as compared to neighboring participants not employing antibiotic supplemented feed. Multiple resistance in the bacteria

Table I. Effect Consuming of Antibiotic Supplemented Feeds on the Incidence of Resistant E. coli

Antibacterials	% Resistant			
	Illinois Swine	Illinois Poultry	Illinois Beef	Montana Range Cattle*
Oxytetracycline	89.8	59	49.1	0
Dihydrostreptomycin	93.2	72	50.0	0.6
Ampicillin	52.5	17	13.2	1.3
Neomycin	20.5	0	12.3	0
Sulfamerazine	82.9	21	29.2	0.6

Adapted from: Siegel et al. (5).
*Range cattle, minimally exposed to antibiotics, served as the control.

was noted for both human and animal subjects and linked with the tetracycline plasmid. The animal to human link has been reported in a number of studies. Holmberg et al. (9) summarized 52 outbreaks of salmonella investigated by the Centers for Disease Control from 1971 to 1983 of which food animals were linked with 69% of the outbreaks involving antibiotic resistant salmonella. For 38 outbreaks of confirmed mode or source (Table II), multiply resistant salmonella were involved in 33% of the community based outbreaks, 40% of the nosocomial, and 75% of the outbreaks involving both community and hospital. In addition, it has been estimated that each culture-documented case among human beings may represent as many as 100 undocumented cases (10). Agency participation for these cases was made at the request of the local health officials and therefore the survey was not random. However, the resistant strains displayed a fatality rate 21 times that of antibiotic sensitive strains. O'Brien et al. (10) found that characterization of plasmid DNA from antibiotic resistant salmonella suggests extensive commingling of human and animal bacteria.

Table II. Outbreaks of Salmonellosis Between 1971 and 1983 Reported by CDC

Source	Number of Outbreaks*			% Resistant Strains
	Community	Nosocomial	Both	
Food Animals or Products	7/12	1/2	3/4	61%
Food Services	1/10	0/1	0	9%
Other Sources	0/2	1/2	0	25%
Person to Person	0	2/5	0	40%
			Mean	39.5%
% Resistant Strains	33%	40%	75%	

Adapted from: Holmberg et al. (9)
*Resistant strains/total outbreak for cases of specific source or mode of transmission.

Evidence for the demonstration of the link of subtherapeutic use of antibiotics in animal feeds to severe disease in humans was proposed in the highly publicized Minnesota outbreak involving a multiply resistant Salmonella newport (11). The provision of evidence linking the subtherapeutic use of antibiotics in feeds to human disease was not conclusive and the proof of origin as well as meat samples confirming the source for the S. newport were not clearly established. However, this study clearly points out the risks involved with establishing multiply resistant enteric pathogens which access human food products. This study combines the liberal manner in which antibiotics are used (prescribed or not) by the general public for cold-type symptoms with the onset of a severe disease state in an otherwise benign and common illness. Of the 18 cases investigated, 11 were hospitalized for an average of 8 days and 10 of these were taking antibiotics prior to the onset of salmonellosis. For the single fatality among these cases, the multiply resistant salmonella compromised antibiotic therapy where a systemic salmonella infection occurred.

Salmonella is considered an inherent defect in raw meats and therefore is not considered an adulterant since the ultimate use by the comsumer involves cooking which destroys the organism. Concern that salmonella and other common food borne pathogens may be presenting an increased risk to human health via antibiotic resistance prompted contracted studies recommended by the National Research Council in 1980. Results of these studies (12) showed widespread multiply resistant Salmonella, Campylobacter, Staphylococcus species and other pathogens among livestock on farms, in slaughter houses and on the meat in the U.S. Their transmission to man appears equally evident. Whether the organisms are more virulent has not been shown but certainly they have an advantage when antibiotics are employed to which they are resistant.

As has been discussed, the use of antibiotics selects for resistant organisms in the intestine and while these organisms may not be pathogenic (i.e. - E. coli) they act as reservoirs of resistant plasmids which can be transferred to pathogenic or nonpathogenic organisms alike. Prior to the antibiotic era, was antibiotic resistance as prevalent? Some light has been shed on this question by the work of Hughes and Datta (13). These authors studied the Murray collection of Enterobacteriaceae strains collected from 1917 to 1954. They tested 692 strains from 433 isolates of which almost all were from human infections. Nineteen percent of the strains contained conjugative plasmids but none of the plasmids showed antibiotic resistance. This work strongly indicates that the mass emergence of resistant strains is a product of the antibiotic era.

Residual antibiotics. With the widespread use of antibiotics in feeds the occurrence of residuals in milk, meat and eggs becomes inevitable. These residuals result primarily from failure by the producer to adhere to adequate withdrawal periods following the use of the antibiotics. In a review by Katz (3), residual antibiotics were found in all animal species marketed in 1976 - 1978.

The lowest incidence of violative residuals were found in poultry and cattle, with swine and calves having the highest.

Antibiotics in milk result primarily from failure to withhold milk from the market after therapeutic treatment of mastitic or otherwise diseased animals. The exposure to antibiotic residuals in food products is an uncontrolled and involuntary situation. Ingestion of these admittedly low dose levels has been of concern due to potential for sensitization and/or allergic reaction to the antibiotic (14). About 10% of the general population exhibit an adverse reaction to penicillin (15). The possibility of primary sensitization to antibiotics via food products, specifically from penicillin in milk, was essentially ruled out by Dewdney and Edwards (16). Their conclusion rests on the improbability of the low levels encountered in milk (0.01 microgram/ml) as being capable of sensitizing an individual. However, in view of evidence that low dose immunization can favor antibody production (17), these residual levels could be capable of sensitization (3). Upon sensitization the dose required to elicit an allergic reaction is highly dependent upon the individual but may be as little as 40 IU (0.024 mg) in a highly sensitized person. Dewdney and Edwards (16) cite the paucity of cases in the literature to warrant the concern given to penicillin residues in milk and question the validity of those that are. However, given the widespread use and misuse of penicillin and the potential for reaction in the above estimated 10% of the population, continued concern appears warranted.

Antibiotics in milk can affect dramatically the production of fermented dairy products such as cheese, yogurt, buttermilk and sour cream. Routine application of antibiotic test kits such as the Delvo kit are required to avoid major losses on the line. Many of the organisms employed are extremely sensitive to antibiotic residuals in the milk. As shown in Table III, as little as 0.05 to 1.0 IU/ml of penicillin and 0.05 to 10.0 microgram/ml of aureomycin inhibited the growth of 19 cheese starter cultures (18). Lower levels are capable of affecting the flavor and texture properties of the product (14, 19) as well as promoting the growth of undesirable antibiotic resistant coliforms (14, 20).

Benefits of Antibiotics

Modern methods of livestock production are intensive and the environmental conditions stress the animals. The use of antibiotics promotes growth and protects the animals from otherwise certain infection under these conditions. Antibiotic-like compounds formed in lactic acid fermentations prevent proliferation of spoilage and pathogenic microorganisms and increase the shelf life of the products. Nisin is a antimicrobial produced by a lactic acid bacterium and is used in some countries as a food preservative. Some lactic acid bacteria are capable of favorably influencing the fecal flora in man and animals.

Livestock production. The growth promoting attributes of antibiotics in feeds reside in their antibacterial activity in the

Table III. Minimum Inhibitory Levels of Penicillin and Aureomycin for Common Dairy Starter Cultures[1]

Cultures	Penicillin U/ml	Aureomycin μg/ml
Lactobacillus lactis A	0.05	1.0
Lactobacillus lactis B	0.05	1.0
Lactobacillus lactis VI04	0.05	3.0
Lactobacillus lactis 431	0.30	0.5
Lactobacillus lactis kw	0.30	1.0
Lactobacillus lactis V109	0.05	0.3
Lactobacillus lactis, myc	0.05	1.0
Lactobacillus bulgaricus 488	0.10	3.0
Lactobacillus bulgaricus 444	0.10	5.0
Lactobacillus bulgaricus R	0.30	3.0
Lactobacillus bulgaricus V71	0.20	2.0
Lactobacillus bulgaricus V12	0.05	0.3
S and R[2]	1.00	10.0
Streptococcus thermophilus H	0.05	0.3
Streptococcus thermophilus T	0.05	0.3
Streptococcus lactis 9	0.05	0.05
Lactobacillus casei	0.05	0.05
Streptococcus durans	0.10	0.2
Micrococcus 8406	0.05	0.05

[1]Adapted from: Shahani and Harper (18).
[2]Commercial Mixed Culture Containing L. lactis and L. bulgaricus.

intestine. This is corroborated by the lack of improvement in growth of germ-free chicks fed antibiotic supplemented feed (21). The improvement in growth is probably a combined effect of the antibiotic on the flora and the small intestine. Antibiotic fed chicks showed histological changes in the intestine similar to those for germ-free chicks as well as shorter and thinner walled intestines. Nutrient uptake is believed to be enhanced by these changes (3). In ruminants, growth promotion is due to increased propionate producing bacteria by selective inhibition of competing flora, decreased microbial protein, decreased rumen solids and dilution rate and increased metabolizability (not digestibility) (2). Other contributing factors may be suppression of mild but unrecognized infections, reduced microbial destruction of essential nutrients, reduced microbial toxins and synthesis of vitamins or other growth promoting factors which become available subsequently to the animal.

Naturally occurring antibiotics in foods. Lactic acid producing bacteria have been selected historically for food preservation in fermented foods such as sausage, cheese, yogurt, sauerkraut etc. Their principle mode of antibiosis is through the rapid production of organic acid (mainly lactic) and the associated lowering of the pH. Other metabolites such as hydrogen peroxide also have been recognized as factors in the prevention of spoilage of fermented products. The consistent use of high numbers of lactic acid bacteria in fermented meats provides for a rapid fermentation which precludes the proliferation of pathogens such as

Staphylococcus aureus, Salmonella spp. and Clostridium botulinum (22). In the case of the latter, the combination of lactic starter with either sucrose or dextrose has proven effective in preventing toxin production even without nitrite (23, 24). Table IV illustrates the inhibitory effect of lactic cultures on the growth and production of enterotoxin by staphylococci in dry sausage (25).

Table IV. Inhibition of Pathogenic Staphylococci by Lactic Cultures in Sausage

Sausage formulation	Storage, 3 da			Storage, 7 da		
	Log CFU	pH	Toxin	Log CFU	pH	Toxin
Without lactic starter	8.84	5.9	+	8.88	5.7	+
With lactic starter	6.78	5.6	−	7.53	5.3	−

Adapted from: Niskanen and Nurmi (25)

The provision of lactobacilli as therapy for acute diarrhea brought on by enteropathogenic E. coli (EEC) has been demonstrated in vitro and in vivo (26). Gilliland and Speck (27) found a high degree of inhibition of Salmonella typhimurium, Staphylococcus aureus and EEC when grown in associative culture with Lactobacillus acidophilus (Table V); they attributed the inhibitory action to lactic acid, hydrogen peroxide and other inhibitory compounds. The inhibitory compounds have been studied further and isolated (28 - 38). They are listed in Table VI. The production of these antibiotics generally required specific media and growth conditions. Recent work in our laboratory investigated the effect of L. acidophilus on Staphylococcus aureus under yogurt production conditons (39). We found the inhibition due to the acid. Hydrogen peroxide production did not account for the total inhibition observed in the yogurt.

Table V. Inhibition of Pathogens by L. acidophilus in Associative Culture

Test Culture	Treatment	Pathogen (CFU/ml)	Inhibition (%)
S. aureus	Control	1.5×10^7	98.2
	L. acidophilus	2.7×10^5	
S. typhimurium	Control	1.7×10^6	86.5
	L. acidophilus	2.3×10^5	
E. coli	Control	3.3×10^7	87.0
	L. acidophilus	4.3×10^6	

Adapted from: Gilliland and Speck (27)

Shahani and coworkers (29, 34, 40, 41) studied acidophilin and bulgarican from specific strains of L. acidophilus and L. bulgaricus, respectively. These compounds were of low molecular weight and demonstrated a wide range of activity against gram negative and gram positive organisms. Table VII shows the results

Table VI. Natural Antibiotics Produced by Lactic Cultures

Culture	Compound	Reference
Lactobacillus acidophilus	Acidolin	(28)
	Acidophilin	(29)
	Lactocidin	(30)
Lactobacillus brevis	Lactobacillin (H_2O_2)	(31-32)
	Lactobrevin	(33)
Lactobacillus bulgaricus	Bulgarican	(34)
Lactobacillus plantarum	Lactolin	(35)
Streptococcus cremoris	Diplococcin	(36)
Streptococcus lactis	Nisin	(37-38)

Table VII. In Vitro Antibacterial Spectrum of Acidophilin[1]

No.	Test Organism	Strain	IC_{50}[2] ($\mu g/ml$)
1	Bacillus subtilis	ATCC 6633	30
2	Bacillus cereus	Difco 902072	29
3	Bacillus stearothermophilus	ATCC 7954	43
4	Streptococcus faecalis	ATCC 8043	45
5	Streptococcus faecalis var. liquefaciens	ATCC 4532	42
6	Streptococcus lactis	NUC	30
7	Lactobacillus lactis	LY-3 France	40
8	Lactobacillus casei	ATCC 7469	42
9	Lactobacillus plantarum	ATCC 8014	60
10	Lactobacillus leichmannii	ATCC 7830	59
11	Sarcina lutea	ATCC 9341	30
12	Serratia marcescens	NU	29
13	Proteus vulgaris	NU	32
14	Escherchia coli	NU	32
15	Salmonella typhosa	ATCC 167	30
16	Salmonella schottmulleri	ATCC 417	30
17	Shigella dysenteriae	ATCC 934	30
18	Staphylococcus aureus	NU (coagulase + ve)	50
19	Staphylococcus aureus	Phage 80/81	60
20	Klebsiella pneumoniae	ATCC 9997	60
21	Vibrio comma	ATCC 9459	30

[1]Adapted from: Kilara and Shahani (41).
[2]IC_{50} = concentration inhibiting 50% of growth.

of in vitro antibacterial activity for acidophilin against pathogenic and nonpathogenic organisms (41). Beyond the potential product stability against pathogens imparted by these compounds, the possible health benefits to the consumer have not been shown.

Nisin is an antimicrobial elaborated by Streptococcus lactis N. Due to the fact that nisin is not used for human or animal therapy or as a feed additive and growth promotor, its use in food is permitted in over 35 countries (42). Little or no definitive information is available concerning the probability of the development of cross-resistance between nisin and other medically important antibiotics. However, use of nisin is not permitted for food in the U.S. or Canada. Nisin is not inhibitory to yeasts, fungi, or gram negative organisms but is active against several gram positive streptococci, lactobacilli, clostridia, staphylococci and bacilli (43, 44). For successful application of nisin to a food product, Hurst (42) suggests that the food be acidic and that the spoilage organims of concern be gram positive. Nisin was first used effectively to prevent gas defects caused by Clostridium butyricum in Swiss cheese (45). The use of nisin as a potential adjunct to or replacement of nitrite in simulated hams was suggested by Rayman et al. (46). These investigators found that due to an additive effect, the nitrite level could be reduced from 150 ppm to 40 ppm while retaining color stability and preservation qualities. However, they reported also the instability of the nisin after storage at low temperatures followed by temperature abuse. The higher levels of nisin needed to compensate for these factors may make this use uneconomical according to Hurst (42).

Natamycin (Pimaricin) has been approved for use on the surface of cheese and cheese slices for mold inhibition (47). Shahani (48) found that natamycin treated cheeses inoculated with toxigenic molds effectively prolonged the shelf life.

Summary

The widespread use of antibiotics in current livestock production methods offers clear cut advantages in terms of growth and efficiency. However, in view of the increased incidence of multiple antibiotic resistant organisms in the food products, the risks imparted by resistant food borne pathogens is of concern to human health. The routes of transfer are varied and may result from routine farm contact with animals and feed, direct transfer from animal to man, or be as complex as transfer from manure to plant flora to man or animal. Evidence of this last mentioned route has been presented by Levy (49). The sheer volume of largely unmanaged or untreated fecal material generated from livestock production virtually assures transfer to humans. By comparison, human use of antibiotics is estimated at less than 1% of animal use, with animals producing manure at a rate up to 400 times that of man (1). Nonetheless, restrictions on the subtherapeutic use of antibiotics in feeds should be met with an equal scrutiny of human therapeutic abuse. Liberal prescribing of these valuable drugs, largely to prevent secondary bacterial infections following viral cold-type infections, is a useless remedy and serves to exacerbate the human health question concerning infections involving resistant organisms. That resistant pathogens may complicate human therapeutic application is a fact. These resistant organisms threaten application of antibiotics deemed vital in human treatment.

The course that industry and government set must balance food production objectives with long term public health considerations. More prudent use of antibiotics in the feed industry as well as in human medicinal practice is required in order to effectively reserve antibiotics for the treatment of serious microbial disease in humans. The human microflora can be influenced effectively by ingestion of lactobacilli. Work in our laboratory has shown a severe reduction of coliforms in the human stool by lactobacilli. These organisms present a highly competative environment for salmonella and other pathogens. Lactobacilli have a stabilizing effect on the intestinal flora and, if used with proper consideration, could act to prevent shifts in the intestinal microflora that favor disease from resistant pathogens. This application could find a role in controlling the buildup of antibiotic resistant organisms in farm personnel who are routinely in contact with antibiotic supplemented feeds.

Research on antibiotics which do not produce multiple resistance is, of course, desirable. Nisin appears to present just such a situation although its applications are narrow. Some feed additives are capable of "curing" multiple resistance in enterics (50). This area deserves more research and emphasis.

Literature Cited

1. Levy, S. B. N. Engl. J. Med. 1984, 311(10), 663-665.

2. Armstrong, D. G. In "Antimicrobials and Agriculture"; Woodbine, M., Ed.; Butterworths: London, 1984; p. 31.

3. Katz, S. E. In "Antimicrobials in Foods", Brannen, A. L. and Davidson, P. M., Eds.; Marcel Dekker, Inc.: New York, 1983; p. 353.

4. Smith, H. W.; Crabb, W. E. Vet. Rec. 1957, 69, 24-30.

5. Siegel, D.; Huber, W. G.; Enloe, F. Antimicrob. Agents Chemother. 1974, 6(6), 697-701.

6. Levy, S. B.; Fitzgerald, G. B.; Macone, A. B. N. Engl. J. Med. 1976, 295(11), 583-588.

7. Wanatabe, T. Bacteriol. Rev. 1963, 27, 87-115.

8. Anderson, E. S.; Lewis, M. J. Nature 1965, 206, 579-583.

9. Holmberg, S. D.; Wells, J. G.; Cohen, M. L. Science 1984, 225, 833-835.

10. O'Brien, T. F.; Hopkins, J. D.; Gilleece, E. S.; Medeiros, A. A.; Kent, R. L.; Blackburn, B. O.; Holmes, M. B.; Reardon, J. P.; Vergeront, J. M.; Schell, W. L.; Christenson, E.; Bisset, M. L.; Morse, E. V. N. Engl. J. Med. 1982, 307(1), 1-6.

11. Holmberg, S. D.; Osterholm, M. T.; Senger, K. A.; Cohen, M. L. N. Engl. J. Med. 1984, 311(10), 617-622.

12. "Report on the Status of the Food and Drug Administration s Proposed Withdrawal of Approvals for Low Level uses of Penicillin and Tetracyclines in Animal Feeds," Subcommittee on Agriculture, Rural Development and Related Agencies, 1985.

13. Hughes, V. M.; Datta, N. Nature 1983, 302, 725-726.

14. Mol, H. "Antibiotics in Milk", A. A. Balkema: Rotterdam, 1975.

15. Atkinson, N. F. In "The Effects on Human Health of Subtherapeutic Use of Antimicrobials in Animal Feeds," National Academy of Sciences, Washington, D.C., 1980.

16. Dewdney, J. M.; Edwards, R. G. In "Antimicrobials and Agriculture"; Woodbine, M., Ed; Butterworths: London, 1984, p. 457.

17. Marsh, D. G. In "The Antigens"; Sela, M., Ed.; Academic: New York, 1975; Vol. 3.

18. Shahani, K. M.; Harper, W. J. Milk Prod. J. 1958, 49, 15-16, 53-54.

19. Hunter, G. J. E. J. Dairy Res. 1949, 16, 235-241.

20. Kastli, P. Schweiz. Arch. Tierheilk. 1948, 90, 685-695.

21. Coates, M. E. In "Growth in Animals"; Lawrence, T. L. J., Ed.; Butterworths: London, 1980; p. 175.

22. Dacus, J. N.; Brown, W. L. Food Technol. 1981, 35, 74-78.

23. Christiansen, L. N.; Tompkin, R. B.; Shaparis, A. B.; Johnston, R. W.; Kautler, D. A. J. Food Sci. 1975, 40, 488-490.

24. Tanaka, N.; Traisman, E.; Lee, M. H.; Cassens, R. G.; Foster, E. M. J. Food Protection 1980, 43, 450-457.

25. Niskanen, A.; Nurmi, E. Appl. Microbiol. 1976, 34, 11-20.

26. Sandine, W. E.; Muralidhara, K. S.; Elliker, P. R.; England, D. C. J. Milk Food Technol. 1972, 35(12), 691-702.

27. Gilliland, S. E.; Speck, M. L. J. Food Protection 1977, 40, 820-823.

28. Hamdan, I. Y.; Mikolajcik, E. M. J. Antibiotics 1974, 27, 631-636.

29. Shahani, K. M.; Vakil, J. R.; Kilara, A. Cult. Dairy Prod. J. 1977, 11(4), 14-17.

linking the subtherapeutic use of antibiotics in animals to the development of serious disease in humans. Notable among them was the work by Thomas O'Brien and collegues the results of which were published in the New England Journal of Medicine in 1982 (13). This study provided for methodology developments that allowed one to determine whether or not plasmids from different sources (man and animal) were identical or similar.

The Center's belief that the continued unrestricted subtherapeutic use of these antibiotics presents risks to human and animal health is based upon consideration of a number of factors:

-- Long-term, low-level feeding of penicillin and the tetracyclines promotes, by natural selection from the pool of normal intestinal flora, those enteric (gut) bacteria that contain R-plasmids. R-plasmids, also known as R-factors, are extrachromosomal genetic material which confer antibiotic resistance to host bacteria. These plamids can be transferred between various kinds of bacteria through cell-to-cell contact (conjugation). Simultaneous resistance to several unrelated antibiotics is commonly carried on a single plasmid and therefore is simultaneously transferred from one bacterium to another.
-- E. Coli strains bearing R-plasmids can be transferred from animal to man. Under the proper circumstances, organisms of animal origin can colonize in the human gut. However, colonization is not considered necessary for transfer of drug resistance to strains that inhabit the human gut.
-- Use of penicillin and the tetracyclines also causes selection for pathogenicity factors, that is, disease-causing factors. These factors and drug resistance have been shown to be linked on the same plasmid. Pathogenicity and antibiotic resistance can therefore be transferred simultaneously to other organisms.
-- R-plasmids can be transferred from normally nonpathogenic E. coli to certain pathogenic strains of bacteria with which they may come in contact in man or animals. Since R-plasmids carry drug resistance, this transfer can result in the creation of pathogenic strains of bacteria which are resistant to antibiotic therapy.

Continued unrestricted subtherapeutic use of antibiotics in animal feed increases the pool of drug-resistant bacteria in our environment. Moreover, the prospect of pathogens becoming drug resistant is, as FDA believes, a real threat to human health.

In a speech before the Congress in 1978, former Commissioner Donald Kennedy stated: "the evidence indicates that enteric microorganisms in animals and man, their R-plasmids, and human pathogens form a linked ecosystem of their own in which action at any one point can affect every other." If the vulnerability of microorganisms to antibiotics is reduced by the use of antibiotics for nonmedical purposes in animals, the effectiveness of medical treatment will be diminished in man. Potential risks to animal health also exist, and while the linkage to human health is indirect, animal agriculture faces the risk directly. The development of resistant strains, which is enhanced by subtherapeutic drug use, reduces the efficacy of those same drugs for the treatment of animal diseases. The overall implications are addressed by Marc Lappe in his book (14), "Germs That Won't Die." He states: "Organisms almost totally resistant to the major antibiotics now run rampant in hospital quarters, nurseries, and animal stockyards alike, creating unprecedented problems for infectious disease control specialists and public health officials. In spite of the awesome nature and speed of this spread of resistant organisms, many American agencies like the Center for Disease Control in Atlanta, Georgia, have only recently recognized the full implications of this problem. Hospitals and physicians (and veterinarians I might add) still only grudgingly admit a problem exists, even as new antibiotics appear to proliferate as fast as the old ones are outstripped by resistant organisms."

NRDC Analysis of Risks to Human Health

On November 20, 1984, Secretary Heckler received from the Natural Resources Defense Council (NRDC) a petition to declare the subtherapeutic uses of penicillin and the tetracyclines in animal feeds an imminent hazard to the public health. NRDC argues that, on the basis of three recently published scientific studies—the O'Brien and the two Holmberg studies discussed earlier—FDA is likely to eventually withdraw approval of the subtherapeutic uses of penicillin and the tetracyclines in animal feeds. NRDC argues, based on these studies, that these uses meet the criteria for imminent hazard under the law. The petition and its impact were discussed before Congress, in hearings before the Committee on Science and Technology in December of 1984 (15).

Before making any recommendation to FDA Commissioner Young and then to Secretary Heckler, the Center for Veterinary Medicine had to evaluate all available information, not just the three studies cited, before deciding on the petition. To assist in identifying pertinent available data and information, FDA decided to hold a legislative-type hearing on January 25, 1985, on the NIH Campus in which interested persons were invited to present their views.

Some 35 individuals representing industry, academia, government, consumers, agriculture, pharmaceutical manufacturers, producers of red meat and poultry, and even a member of Congress spoke either for or against the NRDC imminent hazard proposal. Final comments were due in by February 11, 1985, and an official transcript was prepared.

The criteria used to evaluate the petition were the following:

-- The likelihood that FDA will eventually withdraw approval;
-- The severity of harm pending withdrawal of approval;
-- The likelihood of harm pending withdrawal of approval;
-- The risk to treated animals from suspended marketing; and
-- Other approaches to protect the public health.

The NRDC petition was unique in that it involved an indirect effect, that is, the effect from the use of subtherapeutic levels of penicillin and the tetracyclines in animal feeds on the health of man. Previously submitted "imminent hazard" petitions dealt with direct effects as in the effect of a drug on a treated individual. Because of the indirect effect, demonstration of the harm to man is decidedly more difficult to measure. Quantitation indeed has been one of the major issues since the subtherapeutic use of antibiotics in feeds question arose in the 1950's.

NRDC estimated that between 100 and 300 deaths each year (depending on which of the provided estimates were used) may be attributable to the subtherapeutic use of penicillin and the tetracyclines in animal feeds. In addition, some 270,000 non-fatal cases of salmonellosis may also be due to the subtherapeutic use of antibiotics (penicillin and the tetracyclines) in animal feeds.

NRDC utilized two key rate estimates from the Holmberg paper published in Science during 1984.

A summary of these estimates is as follows:

1. SUMMARY OF THE FIRST ESTIMATE OF MORTALITY RATE:
   a. Approximately 40,000 cases of salmonellosis are reported each year (CDC data base).
   b. 20% to 30% of Salmonella isolated from humans are resistant to one or more antibiotics (CDC data base).
   40,000 cases times 20% due to resistant Salmonella equals 8,000 cases each year caused by resistant Salmonella.
   c. 4.2% death rate associated with resistant Salmonella (from Holmberg, et al.).
   8,000 cases from resistant Salmonella times a 4.2% death rate from resistant Salmonella equals 336 deaths each year from resistant Salmonella.
   d. 69% of reported Salmonella outbreaks due to resistant Salmonella are traceable to animal sources (from Holmberg, et al.).
   336 deaths from resistant Salmonella times 69% traceable to animal sources equals 232 deaths each year from resistant Salmonella associated with animal sources.
   e. 50% of the resistant strains of Salmonella from animal sources result from subtherapeutic use of penicillin and the tetracyclines in animal feeds (NRDC estimate).
   232 deaths from resistant Salmonella from animal sources times 50% of resistant Salmonella from animals due to subtherapeutic use of penicillin and the tetracyclines equals 116 deaths each year attributed to subtherapeutic use of penicillin and the tetracyclines in animal feeds.
2. SUMMARY OF THE SECOND ESTIMATE OF MORTALITY RATE:
   a. 1,000 to 1,500 deaths each year are associated with Salmonella outbreaks (from private communication with CDC).
   b. 76.5% of fatal cases of Salmonella infections are associated with resistant Salmonella (calculated by NRDC from information contained in Holmberg, et al.).
   1,000 deaths from Salmonella times 76.5% of fatal Salmonella infections associated with resistant Salmonella equals 765 deaths each year from resistant Salmonella.

c. 69% of resistant Salmonella outbreaks are traceable to animal sources (from Holmberg, et al.).
　　　　765 deaths from resistant Salmonella times 69% traceable to animal sources equals 528 deaths each year from resistant Salmonella from animal sources.
　　　d. 50% of resistant Salmonella from animals result from subtherapeutic use of penicillin and the tetracyclines in animal feeds (NRDC estimate).
　　　　528 deaths from resistant Salmonella from animal sources times 50% of the resistance in Salmonella from animal sources resulting from subtherapeutic use of penicillin and the tetracyclines in animal feeds equals 264 deaths each year attributed to subtherapeutic use of penicillin and the tetracyclines in animal feeds.
3. SUMMARY OF THE MORBIDITY ESTIMATE:
　　　a. 40,000 cases of Salmonella infections reported each year (CDC data base).
　　　b. 20% of these cases are caused by resistant Salmonella (CDC data base).
　　　　40,000 cases times 20% equals 8,000 cases reported each year caused by resistant Salmonella.
　　　c. 69% of resistant Salmonella outbreaks traceable to animal sources (from Holmberg, et al.).
　　　　8,000 cases from resistant Salmonella times 69% from animal sources equals 5,520 cases reported each year caused by resistant Salmonella attributable to animal sources.
　　　d. 50% of resistant Salmonella from animal sources result from subtherapeutic use of penicillin and the tetracyclines in animal feeds (NRDC estimate).
　　　　5,520 cases times 50% equals 2,760 cases reported each year attributed to use of penicillin and the tetracyclines in animal feeds.
　　　e. 1% of all cases of Salmonella infections are reported (from private communication with CDC).
　　　　2,760 cases times 100 equals 276,000 cases of non-fatal salmonellosis each year that are associated with the subtherapeutic use of penicillin and the tetracyclines in animal feeds.

　　NRDC used Salmonella infections as the model to make their estimates of mortality and morbidity rates. They pointed out that these are conservative estimates (underestimates) because resistance also occurs in other pathogenic bacteria that cause human diseases. Some of the resistance in these other pathogens results from the pool of resistant bacteria in animals, which is ultimately due in large part to subtherapeutic use of penicillin and the tetracyclines in animal feeds.

　　NRDC concluded that there will be no significant negative effect on animal health from banning subtherapeutic uses of penicillin and the tetracyclines in animal feeds. They indicated that the use of these drugs for purposes of improving feed efficiency and weight gain is for economic reasons only and no

Table III. Growth Responses (All in the Same Room) to Penicillin (200 ppm) in the Diet of Chicks 1964-1980*

Year	Number of Experiments	Average Gains Controls	Penicillin
1964	11	250	294
1965	23	289	324
1966	43	291	330
1967	23	267	311
1968	38	262	301
1969	39	266	310
1970	30	271	310
1971	12	316	357
1972	24	193	211
1973	24	183	203
1974	44	189	207
1975	44	188	202
1976	36	190	206
1977	42	235	253
1978	42	230	249
1979	38	255	275
1980	48	245	273

Length of experiments: 1964-1971 -- 19 to 20 days
1972-1980 -- 13 to 15 days

Each experiment contained two replicates of 10 birds each (5 males, 5 females).

*J. Pensack, personal communication.

added to animal feeds as a preventive measure in the control of certain subacute animal diseases.

In the decade of the 1950s, the use of antibiotics in animal feeds led to improvements in animal health and animal production. This contributed to the rise of large units for maintaining meat animals and poultry. These first 10 years should have given ample time for resistant pathogens to have become widespread. Ten years of this spread of resistance ought to have made antibiotics in animal feed useless or deleterious so that their commercial use would cease. Yet this has not happened, even after 35 years. The failure of such a series of events to take place is an unexplained riddle.

One guess is that anaerobic intestinal microorganisms, as yet unidentified, have retained their susceptibility to antibiotics and also, perhaps, that a large reservoir of sensitive wild microorganisms exists as a sort of pool that continually reinfects farm animals and depresses their growth, unless antibiotics are added to the diet.

Most of the research on antibiotics in feeds was from 1950 to 1960, and this led to many interesting findings that have largely been forgotten (4, 5). The diseased conditions that existed on farms before antibiotic feeding was introduced to stop them have not reappeared so that most people today are not familiar with them.

Antibiotic feeding for the control of chronic respiratory disease in poultry was pioneered by White-Stevens and co-workers who used levels of 100 to 200 grams per ton (6). These higher levels became used for treatment of various other infections of poultry, and also for other animals. In pigs, feeds containing 50 to 200 grams per ton are used to prevent or treat bacterial enteritis, leptospirosis and other infections, and in beef cattle against shipping fever and liver abscesses. Obviously, these higher levels include production of the growth effect. Another increase in antibiotic usage came in the 1960s, when a mixture of chlortetracycline, sulfamethazine and penicillin was introduced for addition to pig feeds.

Antibiotics Used at Low Levels in Livestock Feeds

The use of antibiotics at any level in animal feed is strictly regulated by the Center for Veterinary Medicine of the Food and Drug Administration, acting under the US Food, Drug and Cosmetic Act of 1938 as amended in 1958 and 1963 (7). Twelve different antibiotics are approved for use in livestock feeds:

Bacitracin	Oleandomycin
Bambermycins	Penicillin
Erythromycin	Chlortetracycline
Lincomycin	Oxytetracycline
Neomycin	Tylosin
Novobiocin	Virginiamycin.

A level of antibiotic in edible tissues which is judged

safe for human consumption has been set for each antibiotic approved for such use. This tolerance is based on the results of extensive tests for toxicity, birth defects and carcinogenicity. A method of analysis for the drug in animal tissues must be developed by the sponsor of the drug and approved by FDA. Tolerances are measured in uncooked, edible tissues.

A withdrawal time is the time from the last availability of a medicated feed to an animal until its slaughter. This time is set so that the level of residues drops below the lower level of detectability of the antibiotic and is based on a tissue residue study in which animals are dosed with the highest level of drug in the feed for the longest time permitted. The method of analysis must be sufficiently sensitive to detect fractions of a microgram per gram in tissue.

There is an additional protection against residues, because antibiotics in meat tend to be destroyed by cooking., For example, Broquist and Kohler found that chicken breast muscle containing 12 parts per million of chlortetracycline had 0.14 parts per million after roasting at 230° C for 15 minutes and no detectable amounts after half an hour. The original level of 12 ppm was about 60 times as high as would be produced by 400 ppm in the animal feed, without a withdrawal period (8). The UK Swann Committee reported that the only possible effect of residues on consumers arose from penicillin in milk from cows treated for udder infections in which the withdrawal time for the antibiotic had not been observed. Cases of skin rashes were reported from the consumption of such milk by sensitive patients. The Committee commented that "there are no known instances in which harmful effects in human beings have resulted from antibiotic residues in food other than milk" (9).

The question of antibiotics in meat and other edible products was reviewed at length by Katz (10). The USA Inspection and Sampling Program (1973 results) indicated that 5.3% of 529 carcass samples examined for residues of streptomycin, tetracycline, erythromycin, neomycin, oxytetracycline and chlortetracycline were positive; only 17 of 5,301 samples, or 0.32%, were positive for penicillin. The levels of residues that can be expected from feeding subtherapeutic quantities of antibiotics vary with the degree of absorption from the intestinal tract. In chickens, the continuous feeding of 50 to 200 grams of chlortetracycline per ton of feed resulted in residue levels ranging from .036 to 0.11 micrograms per gram of muscle tissue, and from .058 to .199 per gram of liver tissue. These residues disappeared after one day of withdrawal from supplemented feed. The residues were also destroyed by cooking, which was found to destroy all residues of both oxytetracycline and chlortetracycline in the muscle of poultry. The only residues surviving cooking were found in the liver. No penicillin activity was found in the blood, muscle, liver and kidney tissues of broiler chickens or in the eggs of hens fed 100 grams of procaine penicillin per ton. Approximately 98% of the penicillin activity was destroyed in the upper portion of the intestinal tract, and little or no activity reached the small intestine. Katz comments that residues of the tetracyclines in the muscle tissue of animals will not survive normal food preparation procedures, and that "no residues will enter the diet of humans unless the muscle tissue is eaten raw or very rare." Cooking degrades chlortetracycline to isochlortetracycline (11), and oxytetracycline is thought to be converted to alpha and beta apo-oxytetracyclines (10). Katz comments that "the literature contains no data to indicate that either of these compounds has any biological significance."

The widespread occurrence of penicillin sensitivity, and the survival of penicillin residues in meat following cooking, led Katz to point out that "since up to 10% of the population is potentially sensitive to penicillin and its breakdown products, the risk is too great to be ignored," and to warn against injections unless these are carefully controlled. The use of withdrawal procedures should protect consumers against possible sensitivity reactions from penicillin residues.

Resistance

Much of the debate concerning the use of antibiotics in livestock feeds has centered on bacterial resistance. One of the first observations made early in the 1950s, was that the bacterial count in animal feces increased after a temporary decrease when antibiotics, such as tetracyclines, were fed (12). This was in contrast to the effect of sulfonamides, which reduce the count. Obviously, resistance had occurred because the intestinal bacteria were thriving in the presence of antibiotics. Simultaneously, the growth of the animals was increased. Therefore the resistance in itself was not harmful.

The intestine of a warm-blooded vertebrate contains 21 trillion bacteria, many of which have not been identified or grown in test tubes. Many investigators in the 1950s tried to find out the nature of the changes in intestinal bacteria that were produced by feeding antibiotics. The results were variable and often conflicting (4). Some reports have pointed to a decrease in clostridia, but others have not supported these findings. It is certain that the growth response can persist for years in the same animal colony, therefore there must be some type or types of deleterious intestinal microorganisms that do not acquire resistance.

Salmonella

The most serious association of antibiotics with salmonellosis was the 1965 outbreak in England of phage type 29 Salmonella typhimurium, resistant to tetracyclines. Six human deaths were attributed to this epidemic. It was traced to "shotgun" treatment of young calves with antibiotics followed by wide dispersal of the calves (5). Although this epidemic did not involve the use of livestock feeds containing antibiotics, the seriousness of the outbreak led to an inquiry in the UK and a report by the Swann Committee, 1969, into this use. The report of the committee called for a stop to the use of certain common antibiotics in animal feeds in the United Kingdom.

30. Vincent, J. G.; Veomett, R. C.; Riley, R. I. J. Bacteriol. 1959, 78, 477-484.

31. Wheater, D. M.; Hirsch, A.; Mattick, A. T. R. Nature 1951, 168, 659.

32. Wheater, D. M.; Hirsch, A.; Mattick, A. T. R. Nature 1952, 170, 623-624.

33. Kavasnikov, E. I.; Sodenko, V. I. Mikrobiol. Zh. Kyviv. 1967, 29, 146; Dairy Science Ab. 1967, 29, 3972.

34. Reddy, G. V.; Shahani, K. M.; Friend, B. A.; Chandan, R. C. Cult. Dairy Prod. J. 1983, 18(2), 15-19.

35. Kodama, R. J. Antibiotics 1952, 5, 72-74.

36. Davey, G. P.; Richardson, B. C. Appl. Environ. Microbiol. 1981, 41, 84-89.

37. Mattick, A. T. R.; Hirsch, A. Nature 1944, 154, 551-554.

38. Mattick, A. T. R.; Hirsch, A. Lancet 1947, 253, 5-8.

39. Attaie, R.; Whalen, P. J.; Shahani, K. M.; Amer, M. A. "Presented at the 80th Annual Meeting of the American Dairy Science Association", Urbana, IL, 1985.

40. Shahani, K. M.; Vakil, J. R.; Kilara, A. Cult. Dairy Prod. J. 1977, 12(2), 8-11.

41. Kilara, A.; Shahani, K. M. J. Dairy Sci. 1978, 61, 1793-1800.

42. Hurst, A. In "Antimicrobials in Foods"; Branen, A. L.; Davidson, P. M., Eds.; Marcel Dekker, Inc.: New York, 1983; p. 327.

43. Hawley, H. B. Food Manuf. 1957, 32, 370-376.

44. Shahani, K. M. J. Dairy Sci. 1962, 45, 827-832.

45. Hirsch, A. J. Gen. Microbiol. 1951, 5, 208.

46. Rayman, M. K.; Aris, B.; Hurst, A. Appl. Environ. Microbiol. 1981, 375-380.

47. "Federal Register," June 22, 1982.

48. Shahani, K. M. J. Dairy Sci. 1962, 45, 827-832.

49. Levy, S. B. In "Antimicrobials in Agriculture"; Woodbine, M., Ed.; Butterworths: London, 1984; p. 525.

50. Davey, L. A. In "Antimicrobials in Agriculture"; M., Ed.; Butterworths: London, 1984; p. 445.

RECEIVED May 28, 1986

9

Risks to Human Health from the Use of Antibiotics in Animal Feeds

Philip J. Frappaolo

Center for Veterinary Medicine, U.S. Food and Drug Administration, Rockville, MD 20857

Since 1969, the Food and Drug Administration's Center for Veterinary Medicine (formerly the Bureau of Veterinary Medicine) has had cause for concern that the subtherapeutic use of antibiotics in animal feeds may cause bacteria in animals to become resistant to antibiotics. This resistance to antibiotics is said by many knowledgeable scientists to be transferred to bacteria in humans, thus making these antibiotics ineffective in treating human bacterial infections due to compromise of therapy. For this reason, FDA proposed in 1977 to withdraw the use of penicillin in animal feed and restrict the use of the tetracyclines (chlortetracycline and oxytetracycline) to certain uses in animal feed. This talk will focus on FDA's efforts to finalize its review of the issue and present an update on the current status of the 1977 proposals.

In a letter to Science in 1980 (1), U.S. Representative John Dingell (D-MICH) stated with respect to the debate concerning the subtherapeutic use of antibiotics in animal feeds: "The science of this issue is well in hand, but we cannot call upon it to do the impossible. Twenty years of scientific investigation have identified but not quantified the risk to human health. We now face a fork in the road where prudent policy decision and not further study   be the pathfinder."

The   al ways in which the feeding of antibiotics of
                 potential health hazard to humans and other
               hogenic organisms such as Salmonella, existing
                 iimals, can become resistant to the
                 the host animal at subtherapeutic levels and
                 to the environment and/or food to humans.

ter not subject to U.S. copyright.
1986, American Chemical Society

Since the organisms are antibiotic resistant, if they produce clinical infection in humans or other animals, then the same antibiotic would be an ineffective treatment. Secondly, resistance that develops in non-pathogenic bacteria, for example, E. coli may be transferred to pathogenic bacteria either in animals or humans which may in turn cause a drug resistant infection. There is also concern that antibiotics in animal feeds may increase the prevalence or prolong the shedding of Salmonella organisms in animals, thus increasing the risk of disease in animals and humans.

Historical Perspective

The health concerns over the practice of feeding animals antibiotics came to the forefront in 1965 when in England there was an epidemic of drug resistant Salmonella typhimurium in dairy calves that subsequently spread to humans. Thousands of animals as well as seven humans died as a result of the epidemic which lasted for several years. The offending strain of Salmonella was believed to have originated on a calf dealer's premises from which infected calves were sold to many parts of England. The use of antibacterials in the calves was thought to have caused the development of the resistant strain of Salmonella. Spread of the organism and treatment of diseased animals with various antibiotics led to the strain acquiring resistance to eight different drugs by the time the epidemic had run its course.

This incident and concerns that resistance to antibiotics was increasing led to the formation of the Swann Committee, which examined the use of antibacterials in feeds in England. In 1969, the Committee issued its report (2) on the use of antibiotics in veterinary medicine and animal husbandry. It recommended that antibiotics and other antibacterials be divided into a "feed" class and a "therapeutic" class which would be used only by issuance of a veterinary prescription. The British government accepted the Swann Commmttee recommendations in 1971.

FDA's concerns regarding antibiotic resistance and the implications for human and animal health span some 30 years during which symposia, consultations with outside experts and task force reviews were held. Most notable among these actions was the establishment of the FDA Task Force on the Use of Antibiotics in Animal Feeds. Established in 1970 at the recommendation of FDA's Science Advisory Committee, the Task Force was asked to undertake a comprehensive review of the use of antibiotics in animal feeds.

In its report (3) issued in 1972, the Task Force acknowledged the potential human and animal health hazard of drug resistant bacteria and made a number of recommendations. In addition to basic research to better understand the nature of the problem, the Task Force recommended that restrictions be placed on the use of antibacterial agents in feeds which fail to meet guidelines established by the Task Force in regard to safety and/or efficacy. Agents that do not meet these standards would be prohibited from growth promotion and any subtherapeutic use in animals but could continue to be used at therapeutic levels for short-term treatment on the order of licensed veterinarians.

Shortly after the Task Force made its recommendation, FDA in 1973 established a regulation (4) that specified that antibiotics to be used in animal feeds for more than two weeks must meet the Task Force's criteria for safety in order to gain approval or to remain on the market.

A few years after the issuance of the Task Force Report, the Commissioner of the Food and Drug Administration (FDA) ordered additional review of the data and the issues involved by the Agency's National Advisory Food and Drug Committee. This review involved public meetings and comments from all interested parties. After this review and taking into consideration the recommendations of the Advisory Committee, former Commissioner Donald Kennedy directed the Bureau of Veterinary Medicine [now the Center for Veterinary Medicine (CVM)] to publish a Notice of Opportunity for Hearing on a proposal to withdraw approval of New Animal Drug Applications for use of penicillin in animal feeds. This Notice (5) published in the FEDERAL REGISTER on August 30, 1977, and was followed on October 21, 1977, by a similar Notice (6) which proposed withdrawal of certain subtherapeutic uses of the tetracyclines, specifically chlortetracycline and oxytetracycline in animal feeds. The manufacturers of the antibiotics requested a hearing.

Because of disagreement among some scientists as to whether the subtherapeutic use of these antibiotics results in significant health risks, Congress intervened and in 1979 directed FDA to contract with the National Academy of Sciences (NAS) to study the issues involved and earmarked $250,000 for that purpose. Congress also mandated that FDA hold in abeyance any implementation of its proposed actions pending final results of these studies. Nevertheless, FDA announced its intention to hold a formal evidentiary hearing in response to the drug sponsors' request, but the start of the hearing would be delayed until release of the NAS report.

In addition to the NAS report, other Congressionally mandated studies included the Office of Technology Assessment report (7) on "Drugs in Livestock Feed" in June of 1979, and the USDA's report (8) on the "Economic Effects of a Prohibition on the Use of Selected Animal Drugs" in December of 1978. These reports essentially supported the views held by FDA. For example, the OTA report concluded that the health risks from the use of low-level antibiotics are of greater concern than the risks of cancer from DES and furazolidone as used in livestock practice. They also concluded that the drugs FDA proposed restricting could be replaced with alternative drugs. The USDA economic study concluded that while farm and food prices would increase initially, the economic system would generally "be quite resistant to a more restrictive policy on animal drug use." This conclusion was reached even though the USDA study was based on the erroneous assumption that all feed additive antibiotics would be banned.

In March of 1980, the NAS submitted its report (9) entitled "The Effects on Human Health of Subtherapeutic Use of Antimicrobials in Animal Feeds." The report stated "the postulations concerning the hazards to human health that might result from the addition of subtherapeutic antimicrobials to feeds have been neither proven nor disproven. The lack of data linking human illness with subtherapeutic levels of antimicrobials must not be equated with proof that the proposed hazards do not exist. The research necessary to establish and measure a definite risk has not been conducted and, indeed, may not be possible." The NAS committee further concluded that it is not technically feasible to conduct a single comprehensive epidemiological study that will settle the issues. They offered suggestions for several less comprehensive, but more feasible, studies with the caveat that these studies had potential for clarifying certain points, but would not settle the issues. They would, in essence, better define the links in the chain of events that is believed to exist from the feeding of subtherapeutic levels of antibiotics in animals to the development of drug resistant disease in humans.

Recent Events

In view of the NAS report, Congress, through the appropriations process for fiscal 1981, instructed FDA to conduct additional studies to generate new epidemiologic information consistent with the NAS suggestions and hold in abeyance any proposed actions until the studies are concluded. In response to the 1981 mandate of Congress to generate additional data, FDA awarded a contract (10) to the Seattle-King County Department of Public Health to conduct an epidemiologic study of Salmonella and Campylobacter in commercial meat products in the community and their association with human disease. In August of 1984, CVM received the final study report and although it has been accepted as having met contractual obligations, the study is currently undergoing scientific review.

The study used a dual surveillance approach, one monitoring cases of human illness and the other involving the sampling of food for contamination. For human case surveillance, all cases of Salmonella and Campylobacter jejuni enteritis diagnosed in enrollees at Group Health Cooperative of Puget Sound, a 320,000 member health maintenance organization (HMO), were investigated over an 18-20 month period. A case/control study was also conducted. In addition, household environmental samples were taken from family members of index cases, household pets, and in some cases, foods were sampled in an effort to identify reservoirs of Campylobacter. Food surveillance was integrated into the health departments meat inspection program and thus provided access to all retail purveyors of meat products in King County, Washington. Added to the retail meat surveillance system was a specification for culturing poultry products at a large independent poultry processor in Seattle. The food surveillance system was designed to provide for the culture of 2,000 specimens of food products of animal origin for Salmonella and Campylobacter during a 20 month-period. In order to evaluate relationships among individual Campylobacter and Salmonella isolates, antibiotic susceptibility testing was conducted along with serotyping and several types of plasmid analyses.

The predominant finding reported by the contractor in the food surveillance system was significant contamination of retail poultry by Campylobacter jejuni; 22.3% of specimens cultured C. jejuni while only 3.5% cultured Salmonella. The research contractor concluded that enteritis due to Campylobacter jejuni is more common than that due to Salmonella and that C. jejuni appears to flow from chickens to man via consumption of poultry products.

Considerable public attention has been focused on the antibiotics in animal feed issue as of late as a result of two recent reports from investigators at the Centers for Disease Control. One report (11) in the August 24, 1984, issue of Science was a retrospective analysis of all CDC investigated Salmonella outbreaks during the 13 year period between 1971 and 1983. They discovered that in over two-thirds of U.S. outbreaks of miltiple-drug-resistant Salmonella infections that had a defined source, such bacteria came from food animal populations. Animal origins were discovered more commonly in outbreaks involving antimicrobial-resistant Salmonella than in outbreaks involving antimicrobial-sensitive strains. In addition, the case fatality rate for patients with multiple resistant Salmonella infections was found to be 21 times higher than the case fatality rate associated with antimicrobial-sensitive Salmonella infections. Their assessment was that antimicrobial-resistant bacteria frequently arise from food animals and can cause serious infections in humans.

One of the major criticisms of FDA's scientific basis for wanting to restrict the use of antibiotics in animal feeds has been that it has not provided any specific instances of human illness due to drug-resistant pathogens that resulted from the subtherapeutic feeding of antibiotics to animals. However, individual events in the complicated sequence have been documented. Another report (12) by Dr. Scott Holmberg and others at CDC which appeared in the September 6, 1984, issue of the New England Journal of Medicine purportedly linked, for the first time, the use of subtherapeutic antibiotics in livestock feed to the development of serious drug resistant infections in humans.

The article described the investigation of an outbreak of Salmonella newport involving 18 persons in the Midwest. The epidemic strain was resistant to ampicillin, carbenicillin, and tetracycline. Twelve of the patients had been taking penicillin derivatives for other medical problems. Eleven required hospitalization and there was one death. Through epidemiologic techniques ground beef was implicated as the common food source of the infection and the meat was traced to cattle presumably from a farm in South Dakota. The cattle had presumably been fed subtherapeutic levels of chlortetracycline for growth promotion and disease prevention. A major finding in this investigation was the identification of a segment of the population, i.e, those receiving antibiotics, that may be at higher risk of contracting a severe illness due to a resistant Salmonella infection. Presumably, the use of antimicrobials to which a pathogen is resistant would constitute selective pressure permitting the organism to flourish.

There have also been a number of other studies contracted for by FDA since the 1977 notices on the penicillins and the tetracyclines. These studies were designed to provide more information on specific segments in the postulated chain of events health risks to animals will result if these uses are discontinued. The only potential animal health risk involves the use of these drugs for prevention of animal diseases. Since the petition is for suspending uses of penicillin and the tetracyclines, there are other antibiotics that can be used to prevent these diseases. Also, there are effective alternatives to antibiotics, such as vaccines, to prevent diseases. NRDC also advocated changing certain farm management practices, such as reducing the crowding of animals in feedlots, which should reduce stress and transmission of diseases. Both of those actions it was said should reduce the need for disease prevention. NRDC pointed out that it is not advocating a ban of pencillin and the tetracyclines used at therapeutic levels to treat diseases.

NRDC also noted that the frequency of antibiotic resistance in bacteria that cause disease increases when animals are fed subtherapeutic levels of these drugs. Thus, when animals become ill with one of these resistant organisms, treatment with therapeutic levels of the antibiotic of choice may not be effective.

NRDC contended that the suspension of these subtherapeutic uses of penicillin and the tetracyclines in animal feeds poses no human health problem. No potential human health problem has been identified in the literature. Any risk of eating meat from an animal that becomes ill, because penicillin and the tetracyclines were not available, could be alleviated by using substitute antibiotics and better farming practices to prevent or reduce the incidence of disease. Moreover, there would be an increased probability of effectively treating the diseases with therapeutic levels of antibiotics if they were not used at subtherapeutic levels.

According to NRDC, the only possible impact of a ban on humans would be economic. A higher price for meat would be temporary. It was proposed that the average citizen consumes almost three times more meat per year than the U.S. Department of Agriculture considers necessary to meet nutritional needs. Thus, the consumption of a few pounds less meat per person per year because of economic reasons would not have any human health effect according to NRDC.

If the Agency decides to proceed with withdrawal, a formal evidentiary public hearing before an administrative law judge (ALJ) would be required. Under our law, such a hearing would be needed in this case even if the drug uses in question were to be found to be an imminent hazard. Granting an imminent hazard petition does not avoid formal proceedings. Rather, granting a petition suspends the marketing of a drug immediately--before the completion of the formal evidentiary public hearing, the ALJ's initial decision, and the Commissioner's final decision. Under the ordinary withdrawal procedures, in which a drug does not meet statutory requirements but does not present an imminent hazard, the drug may be marketed until the completion of all of these steps.

CONCLUSION

In an article (16) written for the American Journal of Epidemiology, Reuel Stallones, Chairman of the NAS Committee to

Study the Human Health Effects of Subtherapeutic Antibiotic Use in Animal Feeds stated: "Public policy and the actions stemming from it cannot always await the accumulation of scientific evidence and the development of prevailing views among scientists."

At the time of our original proposal to ban the subtherapeutic uses of penicillin and the tetracyclines in animal feeds, the contention was advanced that there were gaps in the scientific position to supporting the chain of events linking low level antibiotic feedings to disease in humans. Since then, newly generated data have been useful in filling these gaps in our knowledge. After FDA reviews and evaluates these new data, the Agency will know whether to proceed with the proposed ban.

In sum, two decisions must be made in the near future. First, whether the hazards to human health are of such significance as to call for an immediate ban of low level uses of penicillin and the tetracyclines in animal feeds, and (2) whether to move forward with the withdrawal proceedings.

CVM is currently engaged in an active review of all available research and other information, particularly that generated since 1977, to assess the impact of this complex scientific issue on the subtherapeutic feeding of antibiotics to animals.

Thank you for allowing me to share these views with you and I am available for any questions that you may have.

Literature Cited

1. Dingell, J., 1980. "Animal Feeds: Effect of Antibiotics" (letter), Science. 208: 1069.
2. Report of the Joint Committee on the Use of Antibiotics in Animal Husbandry and Veterinary Medicine, 1969. Her Majesty's Stationary Office, London.
3. FDA Task Force, 1972. Report to the Commissioner of the Food and Drug Administration on the Use of Antibiotics in Animal Feeds. FDA #72-6008, 23 pp.
4. Code of Federal Regulations, 1985. Antibiotic, Nitrofuran, and Sulfonamide Drugs in the Feed of Animals. Section 558.15: 484-497.
5. FEDERAL REGISTER, 1977. Penicillin: Use in Animal Feed. Vol. 42, No. 168: 43770-43793.
6. FEDERAL REGISTER, 1977. Tetracycline in Animal Feeds and Tetracycline Containing Premixes. Vol. 42, No. 204: 56254-56289.
7. Office of Technology Assessment, 1979. Drugs in Livestock Feed. OTA-F-91, 67 pp.
8. U.S. Department of Agriculture Economics, Statistics, and Cooperatives Service, 1978. Economic Effects of a Prohibition on the Use of Selected Animal Drugs. Agricultural Economic Report #414. IV + 68 pp.
9. Committee to Study the Human Health Effects of Subtherapeutic Antibiotic Use in Animal Feeds, 1980. The Effects on Human Health of Subtherapeutic Use of Antimicrobials in Animal Feeds. ISBN 0-309-03044-7, XVI + 376 pp.
10. FDA Contract #223-81-7041, 1981. Surveillance of the Flow of *Salmonella* and *Campylobacter* in a Community.

11. Holmberg, S. D., J. G. Wells, M. L. Cohen, 1984. Animal-to-Man Transmission of Antimicrobial-Resistant Salmonella: Investigations of U.S. Outbreaks 1971-1983. Science 225-833-835.
12. Holmberg, S. D., M. T. Osterholm, K. A. Senger, ET AL., 1984, Drug-Resistant Salmonella From Animals Fed Antimicrobials. New England Journal of Medicine, 311: 617-622.
13. O'Brien, T. F., J. D. Hopkins, E. S. Gilleece, ET AL., 1982. Molecular Epidemiology of Antibiotic Resistance in Salmonella from Animals and Human Beings in the United States. New England Journal of Medicine. 307:1-6.
14. Lappe, M., 1982. Germs That Won't Die: Medical Consequences of the Misuse of Antibiotics. Anchor Press, Garden City, NY, 246 pp.
15. Committee on Science and Technology: U.S. House of Representatives, 1984. Antibiotic Resistance. 98th Congress, Second Session. Report No. 150, 139-188.
16. Stallones, R. A., Epidemiology and Public Policy: Pro-And-Anti-Biotic, 1982. American Journal of Epidemiology. Vol. 115, No. 4: 485-491.

RECEIVED April 1, 1986

10

Effects of Low Levels of Antibiotics in Livestock Feeds

Thomas H. Jukes

Department of Biophysics and Medical Physics, University of California, Berkeley, CA 94720

> Young vertebrates usually live in a "below-par" condition of subtle ill health caused by unidentified harmful intestinal microorganisms. This is shown by the antibiotic growth effect, in which the unidentified microorganisms are suppressed and by the enhanced growth rate of germ-free chicks and rats, in which the unidentified microorganisms are excluded. When antibiotics are added to the diet of animals, large numbers of resistant enterobacteria become present in their intestines. Resistance is also enhanced by administering antimicrobial drugs to human beings, or to animals by veterinary prescription.
> The outbreak of Salmonella foodborne illness in Illinois in April 1985 was attributed to a tetracycline-resistant strain of Salmonella typhimurium. It evidently had no connection with feeding antibiotics in livestock. The resistant strain was of lower virulence than the average sensitive strain.
> Antibiotics in livestock feeds continue to be effective in promoting growth and suppressing certain diseases of farm animals after more than 33 years of use.

Since about 1952, the American public has been amply supplied with meat produced largely from animals that received feed containing antibiotics. These and other chemicals, including sulfonamides and antiparasitic drugs such as anthelmintics and coccidiostats added to feed, have saved labor, feed and space, thus revolutionizing animal agriculture. The record of safety of antibiotics in animal feed in the US has been excellent, including safety to producers and meat handlers as well as to consumers.

Antibiotics are commonly added to many livestock feeds at "subtherapeutic" levels, defined usually as up to 200 parts per million, commonly expressed as 200 grams per ton. This increases growth and suppresses bacteria that cause certain diseases, some of them subacute. The increase in growth results from an antibacterial effect.

My association with antibiotics in livestock feeds started in 1949 when Dr. Robert Stokstad and I found that aureomycin mash increased the growth of young chickens that received a complete diet., The growth-promoting effect of aureomycin (chlortetracycline) was announced at the American Chemical Society meetings in Philadelphia, April 1950.

The announcement was widely quoted in the press. For example, the Daily Telegraph, London, England, headlined the story, "Drug Speeds Growth 50 p.c.; Effect on Animals," and said that "the American Chemical Society has announced in Philadelphia that the drug aureomycin, hitherto known for its anti-infection properties is also one of the greatest growth-promoting substances ever discovered...and has increased the rate of growth of hogs by as much as 50%." The article also stated that tests were being made with undersized and undernourished children.

So-called normal young animals are in reality slightly sick, and this slows their growth. Their growth is increased by feeding low levels of antibiotics. The response is produced by several different antibiotics that have no similarity either in chemistry or mechanism of action, and whose only common property is that of inhibiting the growth of bacteria. The response may occur in chickens fed antibiotics at levels as low as one gram per ton of feed. Table 1 lists some characteristics of the antibiotic growth effect.

Table I. The Antibiotic Growth Effect

1. Low levels of antibiotics increase growth in healthy animals on nutritionally complete diets.

2. No growth increase by antibiotics in germ-free animals.

3. Duplication by antibiotics of certain physiological effects seen in germ-free animals.

4. Sparing action on nutrient requirement in animals on incomplete diets.

5. Prolonged use of antibiotics on some premises often results in improved growth in unsupplemented animals.

The effect has been observed in animals kept in carefully cleaned surroundings. Sometimes the effect disappears under such conditions, and at other times it persists. For example, the growth effect has been obtained in pigs taken by Caesarean section under aseptic conditions and reared under thoroughly clean, but not sterile, conditions (1).

Antibiotics do not promote growth of sterile, so-called germ-free animals or of chick embryos. This shows that the growth effect is not produced by direct action of antibiotics on animals but results from antibacterial action. Of equal importance is the fact that germ-free animals grow faster than non-germ-free controls. Table 2 shows results by Forbes and co-workers that illustrate these points (2).

Table II. Effect of Antibiotics on Growth of Germ-Free and "Conventional" Turkey Poults*

Status of Turkey Poults	No Supplement		Antibiotics	
	No. of Birds	Weight	No. of Birds	Weight
Germ-free	23	202 g	20	207 g
Conventional	33	170 g	34	212 g
Germ-free	27	201 g	25	199 g
Conventional	37	170 g	36	207 g

*After Forbes et al., 1958, Ref. 2
Six experiments summarized; 14-day weights.
Penicillin, 45 ppm, Oleandomycin, 30 ppm

Conclusions: Growth increase approximately 20% by excluding contamination, or by feeding antibiotic. No effect of antibiotic in absence of contamination.

The effect on growth is highly persistent, and has continued for periods of up to 30 years or more in the same animal colonies, such as at Washington State University, the American Cyanamid Company (Table 3) and the University of Wisconsin. Growth promotion was still obtained with chicks in 1984 at Wisconsin by oxytetracycline and penicillin just as markedly as in 1951 (3).

The growth effect occurs in the presence of resistant intestinal bacteria. One must conclude that in the intestinal tract there are susceptible deleterious bacteria that are inhibited or eliminated, and also there are harmless intestinal bacteria that become resistant. Upon prolonged use of antibiotics in the same animal colony, it has sometimes been found that the control animals grow more rapidly as time goes by in successive experiments, so that the quantitative growth response becomes less, even though it persists. In other cases (3), the response has remained about the same.

The growth response to antibiotics depends on the "disease level," because various subacute diseases in farm animals are controlled by feeding antibiotics. Under these conditions, the growth response is increased, because growth is depressed by such diseases. As a result, subtherapeutic levels of antibiotics are

The Swann Committee report was followed by demands for discontinuing the feed use of penicillin and tetracyclines in the US. These demands were largely based on the claim that transferable resistance was produced by feeding antibiotics, so that genes for resistance in common nonpathogenic organisms, such as Escherichia coli, passed through cell walls to other bacteria, including pathogens. This transfer of genes for resistance can easily be demonstrated in test tube experiments, but transfer evidently occurs less frequently in living animals. The Animal Health Institute has commented that the presence of other materials, such as bile salts and fatty acids, coupled with a very low population of donors in the intestinal tract compared to the trillions of normally present bacteria, minimize the opportunities for conjugation (13).

It was postulated that farm animals that were fed antibiotics could serve as "factories" that produced resistant intestinal bacteria and that the genes for resistance would be spread throughout the environment so that resistant disease would steadily increase. This would make certain common antibiotics useless in treating human diseases. Accordingly, FDA proposed in April 1977 to remove penicillin and tetracyclines from animal feed use and to place them solely on veterinary prescription "for the shortest time necessary to achieve the desired result." FDA said "The theoretical possibility that drug-resistant pathogens can be produced by antibiotic selection has become a real threat with the emergence of human disease (typhoid and childhood meningitis) caused by ampicillin- and chloramphenicol-resistant Salmonella and Haemophilus. The point is that known routes of transfer exist by which antibiotic use in animals contributes to such threats." (Emphasis in original.)

These examples were inappropriate. Overuse of ampicillin in medical practice was discussed by Wescoe on p. 27 of the FDA's own National Advisory Food and Drug Committee Report, on January 24, 1977. Wescoe said (speaking of antibiotics in animal feeds), "I really find it difficult to understand how you believe a hazard exists for instance, relative to Neisseria gonorrheae, where the disease is practically all human, where it has been treated worldwide for many years by ampicillin ... and then strain to say that maybe that is in part due to subtherapeutic doses of the antibiotic in feed." Dr. Wescoe chaired the committee.

Typhoid is treated with chloramphenicol, an antibiotic that is not used in animal feeds. The two illustrations are examples of the fact that resistant human pathogens can result from medical practice.

As a result of FDA's proposals and the need for more information, a committee was appointed by the National Academy of Sciences. Its report (376 pp) was published in 1980 as "The Effects on Human Health of Subtherapeutic Use of Antibiotics in Animal Feeds" (7). The report noted that the use of antimicrobials in animal husbandry has steadily increased since 1950, as has animal production. Antimicrobials are perceived as especially beneficial when animals are being reared under intensive conditions or are being shipped. The committee pointed out that a number of investigators have asserted that low-level feeding of antibiotics to livestock increases the total numbers of bacteria containing resistant plasmids above that resulting from therapeutic veterinary prescribed use and both therapeutic and prophylactic uses in human beings.

If this is true, said the committee, and if these resistant bacteria reach consumers of meat, there would be an increased risk of infection by resistant pathogens, or there would be an increased likelihood of acquiring a nonpathogenic resistant organism that could transmit infectious resistance to pathogens. "Infectious resistance" refers to the transfer of resistant genes between bacterial cells by means of plasmids or episomes. The committee concluded that not enough information was avialable on these issues to determine the effects on human health.

The committee recommended a comparison of subtherapeutic with therapeutic use of antibiotics on the prevalence of resistant transfer factors in meat animals. Also recommended was a study comparing the enteric flora of vegetarians and meat-eaters. A third study would involve workers in abattoirs and their contacts. These studies are in progress under the direction of Dr. Edward Kass at Harvard University and investigators at the Loma Linda Medical School. The committee also recommended further research on the mechanisms of the antibiotic growth effect. The report (7) said there is little indication that sale of antibiotics, including penicillin and tetracyclines, for feed and veterinary use, "has decreased as a result of the Swann Report."

The report (7) summarized work by Richmond and Linton in England who found that 3% of all human prescriptions in a county studied were for tetracyclines, and that sewage from hospitals contained more resistant organisms than did domestic sewage. They concluded that the main selective pressure for tetracycline-resistant organisms was from medical rather than veterinary use. Richmond stated that "no reduction had occurred in the incidence of antibiotic-resistant E. coli in Europe following the implementation of regulations recommended in the Swann Report" (7).

I conclude that the results in Great Britain and other European countries show that banning the use of penicillin and tetracyclines in animal feeds has had no measurable effect on the prevalence of antibiotic resistance, presumably because of the continued use of these antibiotics in human and veterinary practice.

Antibiotics and Salmonella Foodborne Illness

Salmonella are a frequent cause of foodborne illness, commonly termed "food poisoning," going back long before the use of antibiotics. Salmonellosis is of unusual interest and importance to inhabitants of Chicago because of the outbreak starting in March of 1985, caused by a resistant strain of Salmonella typhimurium.

As a result of recommendations made by the National Academy

of Sciences committee that studies be made of the transmission of normal enteric microflora between animals and human beings, a study was undertaken for FDA by the Seattle-King County (SKC) Department of Public Health. FDA decided to fund such a study of the pathogens Salmonella and Campylobacter. The report was submitted and released in August 1984 (14).

C. jejuni caused illness (enteritis) at a rate of 100 per 100,000 persons, 2.5 times as often as Salmonella, and poultry products were contaminated by C. jejuni four times as often as by Salmonella. Food of animal origin from retail outlets was systematically cultured for 20 months, during which time the incidence of enteric illness was monitored among 320,000 members of a local health-maintenance group. Major sources of campylobacteriosis were identified, estimating that almost half the infections came from eating chicken, particularly raw or undercooked chicken. Raw milk, travel to underdeveloped nations, fresh mushrooms, and one outbreak from a single goat dairy were also identified.

The SKC investigators found that beef, pork and turkey were not significant sources of Campylobacter for human beings.

A main finding was the detection in retail poultry of C. jejuni cultured in 192 of 862 specimens examined, as compared with 30 for Salmonella. Other types of retail meat had "negligible contamination by either bacterium." Similarly, 48% of the C. jejuni enteritis cases were estimated to originate in poultry and none in beef or pork. Only a few of the cases were hospitalized. There were no deaths.

The King County surveillance does not show a connection between the use of antibiotics in animal feed and either campylobacteriosis or salmonellosis.

In September 1984, Dr. S. Holmberg and co-workers of the Centers for Disease Control (CDC) reported an outbreak of salmonellosis in 18 patients, 13 of whom had consumed hamburger (15).

The patients carried multiply resistant Salmonella newport. Twelve of them had received treatment with amoxicillin or penicillin. The authors suggest that this "use of antimicrobials to which the S. newport was resistant contributed selective pressure that allowed growth of the organism." A seemingly identical strain of S. newport, as judged by plasmid characteristics, was found following autopsy in tissues of a dairy calf that had died on the dairy farm of one of the patients. The dairy farm was near a beef cattle farm from which hamburger was obtained. Thirteen of the patients had eaten hamburger "from the suspected herd or purchased from markets thought to be supplied with meat from the herd." The authors were informed by the beef farmer that he had added chlortetracycline to the feed for his cattle by hand.

One patient died, and the authors describe this case by saying, "S. newport of animal origin apparently contaminated a sigmoidoscope which may have been inadequately disinfected and eventually resulted in a fatal case of nosocomial salmonellosis."

This patient had severe abdominal injuries following a traumatic accident, following which his spleen was removed.

There are a number of "missing links" in the account. The authors said that "suspect hamburger was not available for culture." Later it was disclosed that nine samples were obtained by Holmberg and were received from South Dakota on April 11, 1983 by CDC. They were examined for the presence of Salmonella. No Salmonella were recovered from any of the specimens, which consisted of six samples of ground beef, two of beef liver and one of swiss steak. These results were obtained by use of the Freedom of Information Act, and were made public in Food Chemical News, June 10, 1985, p. 45. The cattle feed was not analyzed for chlortetracycline.

Publication of the article by Holmberg and co-workers (15) was followed promptly by sensational publicity in the media, especially in USA Today and on television programs. An advertisement by American Broadcasting Company in the New York Daily News and the New York Post invited readers to "watch Burt Wolfe of the Channel 7 Eyewitness News Team as he reveals the frightening side effects we could suffer from the meat we eat," and to tune in November 7 and 8 at 5:00 p.m. to "find out if there's much more in meat--beside fat and cholesterol--that could kill you." As a follow-up to these threats of death by eating meat, ABC, on the next evening, November 9 at 7:00 p.m., aired a coast-to-coast broadcast on the same topic, in which Dr. Scott Holmberg said, in reference to the use of antibiotics in animal feeds, "We are looking at hundreds of thousands of antibiotic-resistant bacterial infections and hundreds of thousands more drug-resistant bacterial infections." The source of these terrifying large statistics was not revealed.

Consumer Reports, March 1985, warned against "licking your fingers while eating raw meat" and said that the findings by Holmberg "appear to pull the rug out from under" those who had claimed there was no link between antibiotics in feed and human disease. The "hundreds of thousands of cases" are not visible in a review of nontyphoidal Salmonella outbreaks between January 1971 and December 1983 (16). Fifty-five Salmonella outbreaks were investigated by CDC in the 12-year period, and, of these, summary reports were available for 52, which affected 3,653 persons, an average of 281 per year. Of these 52 outbreaks, food-producing animals were implicated in 18, and foods such as raw milk and eggs are included, as well as beef, among sources of infection.

The outbreaks described are confined to those investigated by CDC at the request of state health departments and therefore "are not a random sample of all Salmonella oubreaks." However, it is of interest to compare the number of affected persons, 281 per year in the outbreaks studied, with the annual production of 4.2 billion pounds of hamburger in the US, 1982 and 1983. Much of this beef was produced with the aid of antibiotics.

The Illinois Outbreak, 1985

When the Salmonella outbreak occurred in Chicago in March and April 1985, Dr. Holmberg was quoted as saying, "We really only understand two things. The outbreak is causing severe human illness and the Salmonella is a drug resistant variety coming from the general animal population." He also said that he thought the bacteria most likely originated from a dairy herd, and that "the public must now consider the issue of antibiotics in animal feed."

On May 25, Wallace's Farmer reported that the most recent count in this epidemic, which was the largest in US history, totaled over 14,000 confirmed cases and two deaths linked to Salmonella poisoning (17). This is a mortality rate of 0.014%.

According to Holmberg's summary of salmonellosis published in 1984 and covering the years 1971 to 1983, 17 outbreaks involved resistant organisms and affected 312 persons, 13 of whom (4.2%) died from salmonellosis. Nineteen outbreaks caused by nonresistant organisms resulted in only 4 (0.2%) fatalities in 1,912 ill persons. These percentages have been widely publicized. A fatality of 0.26% was reported in 1972 in a report to FDA by a task force (18).

Holmberg's mortality rate of 0.2% for sensitive Salmonella would have produced 28 deaths in the Illinois outbreak of 14,000 cases. His mortality rate of 4.2% for resistant Salmonella would have led to 588 deaths in the Illinois outbreak, 1985. Clearly the resistant strain in the Illinois outbreak was less virulent than the average sensitive strain. Clearly, we can breathe more freely about antibiotics in livestock feeds, in spite of the "media blitz."

The Illinois outbreak in 1985 involved 16,284 cases with two deaths verified as infections from the tetracycline-resistant strain (0.012% mortality) (Final Task Force Report, Salmonellosis outbreak, Hillfarm Dairy, Melrose Park, IL, September 1985). Using the "CDC rates," there should have been 684 deaths from antibiotic-resistant infections, and 34 deaths from infections with sensitive strains.

Is Resistance Increasing?

It has repeatedly been shown that penicillin and tetracyclines retain their growth-promoting activity when used in the same agricultural surroundings for periods of 30 years or longer. Furthermore, tetracyclines continue to be effective in the treatment of both human and animal diseases. Atkinson and Lorian (19) found that E. coli, Staphylococcus aureus, Klebsiella pneumoniae, and Staph. epidermidis showed "virtually the same susceptibilities" to tetracycline in 242 US hospitals, 1971 to 1982.

They examined the proposal that bacterial resistance to antimicrobials is increasing worldwide at an alarming pace. They obtained data that included over 43 million individual tests. The study (19), showed that the resistance of most bacteria to most antibiotics had not changed during the past 12 years. Lorian concluded that any general increase of bacterial resistance was a myth. Many individual cases of resistance are reported in the scientific literature, and this attracts attention, but these cases do not represent a general trend. The opponents of antibiotics in feeds tended to question Lorian's findings rather than adjust their own conclusions to revealed facts.

Animal Welfare and Antibiotics in Livestock Feeds

It has been claimed by some members of the animal rights movement that antibiotics should be banned from use in feeds. One statement was: "In the early 1900s, farm animals were raised on extensive farms, where there was plenty of land, fresh air, and room for animals to respond to their own biological needs. Not only were the farm animals healthy, but the farms themselves were healthy as vital enterprises." (20). This author continued by alleging that the use of antibiotics was not in the best interests of the animals because "agri-business farmers must increasingly rely upon antibiotics [which creates] ...unnatural conditions." I doubt whether she was aware of the actual conditions among animals in "the early 1900s." The land was often contaminated by parasites that caused animal diseases. The fresh air was often so fresh that the animals froze to death. However, I was present when antibiotics were introduced into feeds on farms. It was at a time, in 1950, when bloody diarrhea caused obvious suffering and death in young pigs, when chickens died in thousands, suffocated by air-sac disease, and baby calves perished from scours. These various forms of acute distress were rapidly alleviated by antibiotics. The diseases preceded the use of antibiotics.

The Swann Committee noted that "disease is one of the principal causes of suffering in animals, and in all types of animals the use of antibiotics to control infection reduced the suffering and makes an important contribution to animal welfare" (9). It is indeed ironical that the American Humane Society wants to stop animals from being protected against disease and suffering.

My only interpretation is that the animal rights protagonists don't know anything about farming. This is the most charitable explanation.

Effects on Children

Although the topic is not included in the title of this paper, mention should be made of the effects of low level feeding of antibiotics to infants and children. This was investigated extensively in the 1950s, especially in disadvantaged children in developing countries where diarrhea and fecalism are common, just as in young farm animals. The effects were predominantly beneficial and no problems with resistance were reported (5). Recently the use of oral rehydration salts with penicillin has been described by UNICEF (21).

Discussion

There are three main arguments or theories against the use of low levels of antibiotics in livestock feeds. The first theory says

Drugs are used in agriculture to promote growth, improve feed efficiency and to control disease. Modern methods of producing animal-derived food depend heavily on the use of antibacterial substances. In discussing the regulatory concerns for antibiotics in agriculture, one needs to review how tolerances have been established for drug residues in animal products. Table 1 gives the

TABLE I. DEFINITIONS OF TOLERANCES AND TOXICITY TESTS FOR REQUESTED TOLERANCE WITH SAFETY FACTORS

Tolerance	Definition	Toxicity test required	Safety factors
Negligible tolerance*	Toxicologically insignificant residue	90-Day subacute study in rat and dog (preferably in utero for rat)	2,000
Finite tolerance	Measureable amount of residue	Lifetime studies in rat and mouse; 6-month study in dog; 3-generation reproduction study with teratologic phase	100+

* - Residue must be < 0.1 ppm in meat and < 10 ppb in milk and eggs.
+ - If teratogenic activity is demonstrated, the safety factor is 1,000; may also be < 100 when human exposure data are available or when a sensitive measurement is used to set a no-effect concentration.

definition of two types of tolerances that have been used in regulating animal drugs since 1966. A negligible tolerance has a value of 0.1 part per million (ppm) in meat. Negligible tolerances were obtained by drug sponsors by conducting two ninety-day subacute studies generally one in the rat and one in the dog. A safety factor of 2000 was used to calculate tolerances based on these two studies. If the calculated tolerance exceeded 0.1 ppm, the tolerance was arbitrarily set at 0.1 ppm; consequently, most antibiotics have tolerances of 0.1 ppm. If a sponsor desired a higher tolerance than 0.1 ppm, additional toxicological studies were required. To obtain a finite tolerance, that is a tolerance above 0.1 ppm, lifetime studies in the rat and mouse were required; in addition, a six month study in the dog and a three generation reproduction study with a teratological phase were also required. Because of the chronic nature of these studies, the safety factor was reduced from 2000 to 100.

The equation for calculating a tolerance based upon the toxicity studies is presented in Table 2. The various toxicity studies are examined to determine the lowest no-effect level in each of the species. The no-effect level in the most sensitive species is used to determine the tolerance. The tolerance is equal to the no-effect

TABLE II. CALCULATION OF TOLERANCE FOR A DRUG RESIDUE

$$\text{TOLERANCE} = \frac{\text{NEL} \times 60 \text{ KG}}{(\text{SF})(\text{FF})(0.5 \text{ KG/DAY})}$$

NEL = NO-EFFECT LEVEL IN THE MOST SENSITIVE TEST SPECIES

SF = SAFETY FACTOR

FF = FOOD FACTOR

level times the average weight of a person (60 kg) divided by the safety factor, a consumption factor and 0.5 kg, the estimated consumption of meat per day. The consumption factor is an acknowledgement that organ meats, such as liver and kidney, are not consumed to the same extent as muscle tissue. The consumption factors for the various edible products of the different species are given in Table 3. For example, the consumption factor for muscle in all species is

TABLE III. RELATIVE FACTORS FOR ASSIGNING NEGLIGIBLE TOLERANCES MAJOR SPECIES CATEGORIES

Tissue	Beef	Pork	Sheep	Poultry
Muscle	1	1	1	1
Liver	2	3	5	3
Kidney	3	4	5	-*
Skin	-*	4	-*	2
Fat	4	4	5	2

* Not used for human food.

1. The consumption factor for beef liver is 2. Because of this doubling of the consumption factor, the tolerance in liver can be twice the value of the tolerance for the drug in muscle. The consumption factor for pork liver is 3, indicating that pork liver is consumed less than beef liver. Because of these consumption factors, the tolerances in the Code of Federal Regulations (CFR) differ depending on what edible tissue is being described. However, some of the older tolerances in the CFR give the same value for all edible tissues. These drugs were regulated before the use of consumption factors were developed.

The violation rate for antibiotics, as determined by USDA, also needs to be examined in order to discuss the regulatory concerns for antibiotic residues. Table 4 lists the violative residue rates for antibacterials in several species for the years 1979 through 1983.

TABLE IV. VIOLATIVE RESIDUE RATES FOR ANTIBACTERIALS (%)

	1979	1980	1981	1982	1983
MATURE CATTLE	2.2	-	-	-	.2
CHICKENS	nil	-	-	-	nil
TURKEYS	2.4	-	-	-	.01
BOB VEAL	7.8	3.9	7.3	6.1	7.7
SWINE	10	6.8	8.7	7	9.2

The residue violation rate in mature cattle, chickens, and turkeys, is very low, 0.2% or less. In fact, chickens have almost a zero violation rate. This is due to the highly integrated chicken-producing operations in this country, whereas turkeys are raised more by independent producers. However, the violation rate for turkeys is still very low. The violation rate is not low for all species. Bob veal through 1979 to 1983 has had a very large violation rate relative to the other species. This is due to the fact that bob veal are given drugs to keep them alive until they are marketed. As bob veal are marketed as young as 10 days of age, the likelihood of withdrawal periods being followed for bob veal is not high. Some of the drugs used in bob veal require more than 10 days to deplete to below their established tolerances.

The violation rate in swine is also relatively high. This is primarily due to residues of sulfamethazine. The high violation rate for sulfamethazine in swine is due to several factors. Powdered sulfamethazine is electrostatic and tends to adhere to mixing equipment. This effect leads to contamination of nonmedicated feed. Studies indicate that average levels of contamination as high as 3 ppm can occur. These levels in the withdrawal feed of swine can cause violative residue levels. Another problem is in the husbandry of swine. Pigs are coprophagic and as little as 2-3 ppm of sulfamethazine in the feces will also result in violative residues. Compounding the problem has been the refusal of some producers to follow the withdrawal period. A recent publication of USDA indicates that half of the violations of sulfamethazine in swine are the result of producers not following the withdrawal period (1). Based on the conservative nature of the negligible tolerance concept and the low violation rate of antibacterials, the regulatory concern for antibiotics is not large.

The Center for Veterinary Medicine is no longer using the concept of a negligible tolerance in its approval process. The current procedures for calculating tolerances for drug residues have the potential of further reducing our regulatory concern for many of the approved animal drugs. Table 5 lists the minimal toxicological testing for an animal drug by today's standards. These tests essentially replace the studies required to obtain a negligible tolerance, i.e., the two ninety-day feeding studies. The first thing that is required is a battery of genetic toxicity tests to help assess potential carcinogenicity of an animal drug. The second requirement is the

TABLE V. MINIMUM TOXICOLOGICAL TESTING FOR AN ANIMAL DRUG

---

0   A BATTERY OF GENETIC TOXICITY TESTS

0   A 90-DAY FEEDING STUDY BOTH IN A RODENT SPECIES (USUALLY THE RAT)
    AND IN A NON-RODENT MAMMALIAN SPECIES (USUALLY THE DOG).

0   A TWO-GENERATION REPRODUCTION STUDY WITH A TERATOLOGY COMPONENT
    IN RATS.

---

ninety-day feeding studies in both a rodent species, usually the rat and in a non-rodent mammalian species, usually the dog. The third requirement is a two-generation reproduction study with a teratology component in rats. Although the minimum toxicological studies required by today's standards are more extensive, the 0.1 ppm cap for the tolerance has been raised to 1.0 ppm in the total daily diet of an individual. Assuming that one-third of the daily diet is composed of meat products, the 1 ppm in the diet means that a tolerance of up to 3 ppm in the meat can be obtained based on these studies. The 3 ppm is the tolerance in muscle tissue.

Using the consumption factors previously discussed, the tolerance in kidney, liver, and skin/fat can be several multiples higher than 3 ppm. Most drugs that we see in the program today would not require a tolerance higher than 3 ppm because their residue levels are usually much less than 3 ppm in muscle tissue. In fact, several drugs have tissue residues in the ppb range at zero withdrawal. If a drug requires an assigned tolerance greater than 3 ppm to obtain approval, if the residues bioaccumulate, or if it is a suspect carcinogen, additional toxicological tests are required. Table 6 lists

TABLE VI. TOXICOLOGICAL TEST REQUIRED WHEN RESIDUE LEVELS EXCEED
           3PPM, THE DRUG IS A SUSPECT CARCINOGEN, OR THE DRUG IS
                       EXPECTED TO BIOACCUMULATE

---

0   Chronic bioassays for oncogenicity/chronic toxicity in each of
    two rodent species.

0   A chronic bioassay (one year) in a non-rodent mammalian species
    (usually the dog).

0   A teratology study in a second species.

0   Other specialized testing if necessary.

---

the toxicological studies required under these conditions. In addition to the subchronic studies, chronic studies are required in two rodent species and a non-rodent species, usually the dog. Also, a teratology study is required in a second species and depending on specific concerns other specialized testing may be required. A liberalizing aspect of the new toxicological requirements is that the safety factor for subchronic studies has been reduced from 2000 to 1000.

The recent change in the method of calculating tolerances within the animal drug program in CVM will have quite a dramatic effect on the permitted tolerances supported by subchronic studies. Table 7 lists a few representative drugs that are currently regulated in food-producing animals. The first column is the no-effect

TABLE VII. SELECTED ANTIBIOTICS APPROVED FOR USE IN FOOD PRODUCING ANIMALS

Drug	NEL (mg/kg)	CFR Tol. (ppm)	Possible Tol. (ppm)
Apramycin	25	0.1	3.0
Bacitracin (Zn, MD)	>50	0.5	6.0
Erythromycin	25	0.1	3.0
Gentamicin	60	0.1	7.2
Oleandomycin	200	0.15	24.0
Oxytetracycline	365	1.0	438.0
Tylosin	40	0.2	48.0

level for the drug that was used to determine the current tolerance as listed in the CFR. The second column lists the current tolerance. The third column indicates the possible tolerance based upon the formula given in Table 2. Apramycin, for example, would have a possible tolerance of 3 ppm. This is a substantial increase over the present tolerance of 0.1 ppm. Similarily, the current tolerance of 0.5 ppm for bacitracin could possibly be justified as 6 ppm based upon the no-effect level alone. However, current policy would limit the tolerance in muscle to 3 ppm. The tolerance for erythromycin would increase from 0.1 up to 3 ppm. Gentamicin could possibly jump from 0.1 to 7.2, but again would be limited to 3.0 based upon our policy. The no-effect level of the last three drugs listed in the table, oleandomycin, oxytetracycline, and tylosin, indicate the safety of these compounds. These drugs would all be candidates for a revised tolerance of 3 ppm based on conventional toxicity.

These tolerances are not all being automatically revised in the CFR for several reasons: (1) the subchronic studies used to calculate the current tolerances may not meet todays standards, (2) most of these drugs were regulated on the basis of residues of parent drug only, (3) the official methods for monitoring the residues may not meet present standards, and (4) some of the drugs have safety concerns that are not satisfied by subchronic studies.

Present standards require that drugs be regulated on the basis of total residues. Total residues resulting from drug administration to an animal consist of the parent drug and all compounds derived from it, i.e., metabolites, conjugates, and residues bound to biological macromolecules. Total residues are typically determined in all edible tissues by dosing the animal under proposed use conditions with a radiolabeled drug. Several animals are usually employed in such a study to permit their serial sacrifice after the drug has last been administered. From such an experiment, the depletion of total residues in each of the tissues can be followed. Figure 1 represents a typical depletion curve for total residues of a drug. The withdrawal period is approximated by the point in time where the total residue curve intersects the safe concentration level, previously referred to as the tolerance, as determined by the toxicological studies and the formula in Table 2.

To ensure compliance with the withdrawal period, an assay is needed to monitor total residues in the edible tissues. Because it is impractical to develop assays for each residue in each of the edible tissues, the concept of a marker residue and a target tissue is introduced. The marker residue is a selected analyte whose level in a particular tissue has a known relationship to the level of the total residue of toxicological concern in all edible tissues. Therefore, it can be taken as a measure of the total residue of interest in the target animal. The information obtained from studies of the depletion of the radiolabeled total residue can be used to calculate a level of the marker residue that must not be exceeded in a selected tissue (the target tissue) if the total residue of toxicological concern in the edible tissues of the target animal is not to exceed its safe concentration.

In the example depicted in Figure 1, the safe concentration is 2.0 ppm. The marker residue is at a level of 1.0 ppm when the safe concentration is 2.0 ppm. The method is developed for the marker residue at 1.0 ppm and the tolerance for the drug is 1.0 ppm of the marker residue. The overall effect of regulating on total residues as opposed to the parent drug is a lowering of the tolerance. The amount by which the tolerance decreases depends on the proportion of the parent drug to the total residues. For some antibiotics the parent drug is a good approximation of total residues because they are not metabolized. For other drugs the parent drug is a vanishingly small fraction of the total residue and the parent drug would not serve as a marker residue for the total residue. In the latter case, the tolerances would be greatly reduced based upon the low percentage of parent drug. A few of the currently regulated antibiotics would not require total residue studies to support requests for new uses. The tetracyclines are not significantly metabolized and the parent drug is a good approximation of the total residues. We do recognize that degradation to the epi form may occur to a small extent. The aminoglycosides undergo limited metabolism and their absorption from the GI tract is low. Residue studies on gentamicin using microbiological assays, radiotracers and RIA techniques all gave the same results. The lack of absorption also has been demonstrated with the polypeptides bacitracin and bambermycins.

Another reason that the tolerance is not automatically raised in accordance with our new policy, is the question of adequate that this practice turns farm animals into producers of antibiotic resistant genes that spread throughout the environment and convert sensitive pathogens to resistance. I have challenged this theory on the basis of the continued effectiveness of antibiotics in livestock feeds for more than 34 years. The actual results of hospital tests, as reported by Lorian and his co-workers, are also contrary to this theory because these results do not show a general increase in resistance.

The second argument states that resistant salmonellae are more virulent than sensitive salmonellae, and that in consequence the use of antibiotics in animal feeds increases the danger of Salmonella to public health. This theory was given a test in Chicago last spring. The resistant strain of Salmonella was of outstandingly low virulence, less virulent than the average sensitive strain. Lorian has stated that practically all the published work on bacterial virulence and antibiotics "points to the fact that in experiments in animals and the experience in clinical medicine, bacteria that are resistant to one or multiple antibiotics are either equally or less virulent than the nonresistant sensitive organs." Jarolmen and Kemp found that smooth virulent strains of Salmonella acquired resistance much less readily than rough strains that were less virulent for mice (22).

It has been argued (15) that the virulence of infection with resistant Salmonella is heightened if the infected individuals are simultaneously being dosed for colds, etc. with antibiotics, because the antibiotics destroy sensitive nonpathogenic bacteria in the intestine, thus providing more "living space" for resistant Salmonella. But Aserkoff and Bennett (23) found that a course of ampicillin or chloramphenicol prolonged salmonellosis regardless of sensitivity or resistance.

The third argument is that antibiotics in animal feeds, in veterinary prescriptions, and in human prescriptions, all contribute to resistance, and that only the first of these three uses should be discontinued. This argument is challenged by results in Europe. There was no decrease in resistance in E. coli following the ban on penicillin and tetracycline in animal feeds as enacted following the Swann report.

Salmonellosis remains a major public health problem that is reduced by sanitary procedures and adequate cooking. It is not tied to the use of low levels of antibiotics in livestock feeds and it will continue to erupt regardless of antibiotic use.

Literature Cited
1. Hill, E. G.; Larson, N. L. J. Anim. Sci. 1955, 14, 395.
2. Forbes, M.; Supplee, W. C.; Combs, G. R. Proc. Soc. Exptl. Biol. Med. 1958, 99, 110.
3. Dafwang, I. I.; Bird, H. R.; Sunde, M. L. Poultry Sci. 1984, 63, 1027.
4. Jukes, T. H. "Antibiotics in Nutrition"; Medical Encyclopedia Inc.: New York, 1955, 128 pp.

5. Jukes, T. H. Adv. Appl. Microbiol. 1973, 16, 1.
6. White-Stevens, R. H.; Zeibel, H. G.; Walker, N. E. Cereal Sci. 1956, 1, 101.
7. "The Effects on Human Health of Subtherapeutic Use of Antimicrobials in Animal Feeds"; National Academy of Sciences: Washington, D.C., 1980, Office of Publications, NAS, 2102 Constitution Ave., N.W., Washington, D.C., 20418.
8. Broquist, H. P. Kohler, A. R. Antibiotics Annu. 1953:4, 409.
9. Swann, M. M. (Chairman) "Report of Joint Committee on the Use of Antibiotics in Animal Husbandry and Veterinary Medicine"; Her Majesty's Stationery Office: London, 1969.
10. Katz, S. E. "Appendix E: in "The Effects on Human Health of Subtherapeutic Use of Antimicrobials in Animal Feeds"; National Academy of Sciences: Washington, D.C., 1980, Office of Publications, NAS, 2102 Constitution Ave., N.W., Washington, D.C., 20418, pp. 158-181.
11. Shirk, R. J.; Whitehall, A. R.; Hines, L. R. Antibiotics Annual, 1956-1957, Medical Encyclopedia, Inc., N.Y., pp. 843-848, 1957.
12. Johansson, K. R.; Peterson, G. E.; Dick, E.C. J. Nutr. 1953, 49, 135.
13. Issue Briefing Book: "Subtherapeutic Use of Antibiotics in Animal Feeds"; Animal Health Institute: Alexandria, VA 22313, 1985, 30 pp.
14. "Surveillance of the Flow of Salmonella and Campylobacter in a Community"; Communicable Disease Control Section, Seattle-King County Department of Public Health, Seattle, August, 1984.
15. Holmberg, S. D.; Osterholm, M. T.; Senger, K. A.; Cohen, M. L. N. Engl. J. Med. 1984, 311, 617-622.
16. Holmberg, S. D.; Wells, J. G.; Cohen, M. L. Science 1984, 225, 833-835.
17. Wyant, S. Wallaces Farmer 25 May 1985.
18. FDA Task Force "Report to the Commissioner of the Food and Drug Administration: Beltsville, MD."
19. Atkinson, B. A.; Lorian, V. J. Clin. Microbiol. 1984, 20, 791-796.
20. Knopke, M. "Penicillin and Tetracycline Used in Animal Feeds"; Public Hearing 25 January 1985, Food and Drug Administration, pp. 367-374.
21. DeJong, D. UNICEF News 1981, 107, 26.
22. Jarolmen, H.; Kemp, G. A. J. Bacteriol. 1969, 97, 962.
23. Aserkoff, B.; Bennett, J.V. N. Engl. J. Med. 1969, 281, 636-640.

RECEIVED May 28, 1986

RESIDUES

11

Antibiotic Residues in Food: Regulatory Aspects

Robert C. Livingston

Center for Veterinary Medicine, U.S. Food and Drug Administration, Rockville, MD 20857

> The Food and Drug Administration has the responsibility of ensuring that residues of drugs in animal-derived food are safe for human consumption. The permitted residue levels and the conditions of use of each individual drug are determined by toxicological and chemical studies. The studies required for antibiotics vary according to the drug and the proposed application. This paper discusses the following points: (1) the requirements for approval of a new antibiotic as well as those for a new use of an approved antibiotic, (2) the effects of recent changes in the requirements on the amount of residues permitted in food, and (3) deficiencies in current methods for determining antibiotic residues in food.

The Food & Drug Administration has the responsibility for the premarket clearance of all animal drugs. The 1958 food additive amendment to the Federal Food, Drug & Cosmetic Act requires sponsors to demonstrate the safety of their products. The Kefauver-Harris amendment of 1962 requires the sponsors to demonstrate, in addition to safety, the efficacy of their drugs. Safety implies safety to the animal as well as to the consumers of animal products. The role of the Center for Veterinary Medicine in the premarket approval process is to establish conditions of drug use and to establish the allowable tolerances for drug residues in animal-derived food products.

The two major questions concerning the use of antibiotics in agriculture are the safety of the residues in the animal-derived food and the antibiotic resistance that may develop from the use of these drugs in animals. I will not talk about antibiotic resistance as Mr. Frappaolo discusses this issue in a separate paper. The residue issue can be further divided into the toxicity and the allergic reaction to the drug residues. There is sufficient concern for the allergic reaction to penicillin that its tolerance is based upon this concern; however, the rest of the antibiotics have tolerances based on toxicity other than the allergic reaction.

This chapter not subject to U.S. copyright.
Published 1986, American Chemical Society

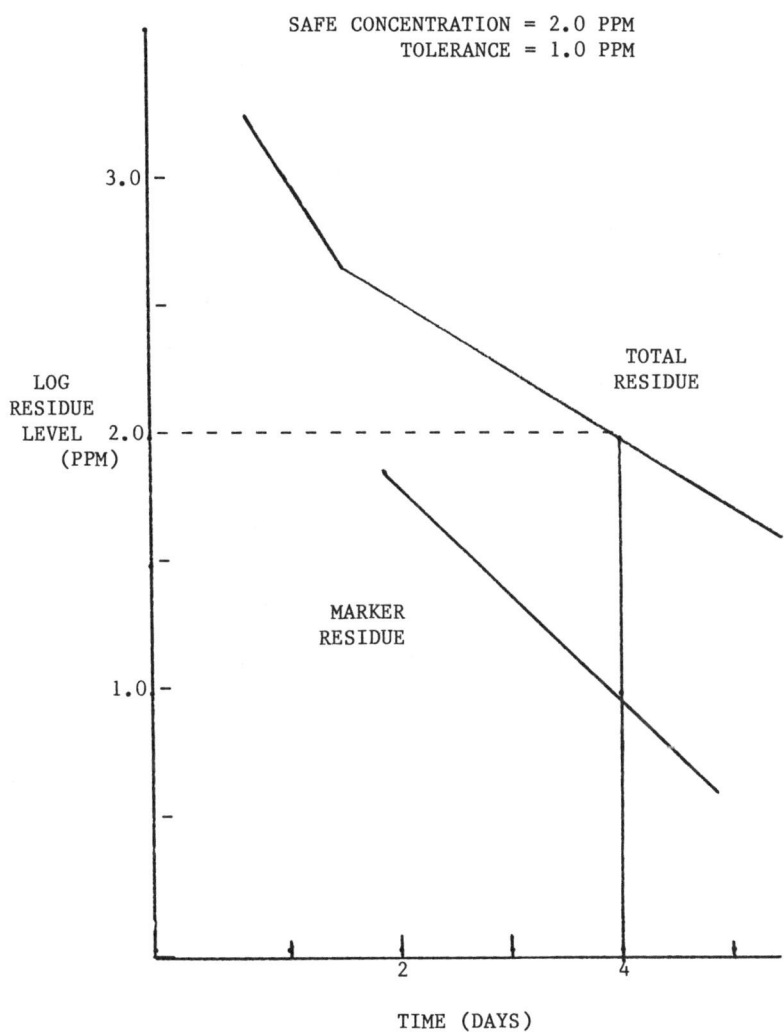

Figure 1. Typical depletion curve for total residues and a marker residue in an edible tissue.

methods to monitor residues. Most of the antibiotics have microbiological assays as methods for monitoring residues. These methods are not specific and are limited to measuring biologically active residues. The adequacy of the extraction procedures for these methods has recently been questioned. If the method does not measure all of the drug residue, the withdrawal periods will be too short. The need for chemical methods for many of the antibiotics was the subject of a recent Association of Official Analytical Chemists symposium.

Sulfamethazine is an example of a drug where the tolerance would not be raised based only on subchronic studies because of its possible carcinogenicity. FDA is presently conducting chronic studies in both rats and mice as well as a total residue study at the National Center for Toxicological Research. These studies are to be completed next year. As the Director of CVM stated in a speech at the Food Editors Conference in Dallas last June, these studies "will either exonerate sulfamethazine or will incriminate it to a point incompatible with continued approval." In either case, the violation problem disappears. In summary, the regulatory concerns for residues of regulated antibiotics is not large. This is due to the conservative procedures for setting most tolerances and the low violation rates. Another reason for the lack of concern of residues of regulated antibiotics is the number of new antibiotics that qualify for zero withdrawal periods. The fact that their relative safety enables them to obtain zero withdrawal periods places competitive pressure on sponsors to also develop safer drugs. There are some specific problems but they are being addressed and the future violation rates should even be lower than present levels.

Literature Cited

1. Fed. Regis. 50: 20796 (May 20, 1985)

RECEIVED June 10, 1986

12

The U.S. Department of Agriculture Meat and Poultry Antibiotic Residue Testing Program

Bernard Schwab[1] and Jeffrey Brown[2]

[1] U.S. Department of Agriculture, Food Safety and Inspection Service, Beltsville, MD 20705
[2] U.S. Department of Agriculture, Food Safety and Inspection Service, Washington, DC 20250

> The USA monitoring and surveillance programs for detecting antibiotic residues in the domestic and imported meat supply are described. An overview of the field/laboratory tests currently in use is also provided.

Antibiotics are used extensively in raising meat animals and poultry in the United States (USA) and other nations. The antimicrobials are used as feed additives or medicants; they allow for faster weight gain and more concentrated rearing practices, and protect the maturing animals against the various diseases that may occur on the farm.

The Food Safety and Inspection Service (FSIS) of the United States Department of Agriculture (USDA) is responsible for providing meat and poultry products to the consumer that are safe, wholesome, and unadulterated. Before marketing, meat animals and poultry must be properly withdrawn from antibiotics to ensure that the levels of antibiotics in edible tissues at slaughter are at or below the tolerances established by the Food and Drug Administration (FDA). FDA is responsible for the approval and regulation of animal drugs used in animal husbandry in the USA. The FDA is also responsible for establishing tolerances for any antibiotics that may adulterate food products and animal feed.

National Residue Program

Since 1967 FSIS has conducted the National Residue Program to help prevent the marketing of animals and poultry containing illegal residues of antibiotics, drugs, and other chemicals.

The National Residue Program operates in three basic modes: monitoring, surveillance, and exploratory.

Monitoring is the random sampling of healthy-appearing animals at slaughter. The data gained from analysis of these samples are

This chapter not subject to U.S. copyright.
Published 1986, American Chemical Society

used to define the profile or residues over time and to identify problems.

Surveillance is biased sampling directed at particular carcasses or products. Surveillance comes into play when the Program receives information from monitoring or other sources, e.g., from slaughter inspection, indicating that adulterating residues may be present. Product may be held until laboratory tests determine the appropriate regulatory action.

Exploratory sampling is done generally to gain information about possible residues of concern. All exploratory projects have in common the negative characteristic that their design is not suitable for immediate regulatory action. However important to the Program, they are basically for informational purposes.

Meat and Poultry products exported to the USA are also checked for antibiotic residues. Imported meat must meet the same residue standards as those established for domestic production. Monitoring, surveillance, and exploratory subprograms as defined above are carried out on foreign production marketed in the USA.

Compound Evaluation and Selection

It is, of course, not feasible to monitor residues of all chemicals that theoretically could contaminate meat and poultry, nor is this necessary to adequately protect public health. It is important, however, to monitor those chemicals that are most likely to present the greatest risk.

FSIS is currently implementing a new prototype system for more refined categorization of residues as to their potential impact on public health. FSIS believes that this Compound Evaluation System (CES) will be sufficiently flexible to permit rapid response to new information that may affect previous rankings and to allow for the use of scientific or expert judgement. As such, the CES should serve as a useful guide in the planning and allocation of FSIS program resources for those residues considered to have the greatest potential effect on public health.

Methods and Testing Program

The effort to reduce the incidence of antibiotic residues in the meat supply involves not only FSIS and FDA, but also the farmers, their trade associations, feed manufacturers, and veterinarians. FSIS has expended considerable resources recently investigating several antibiotic residue problems, such as sulfonamides and antibiotic residues in bob veal calves, and sulfonamides and chloramphenicol in pigs. Agency representatives apprise the industry and other involved parties of the problem and provide resources such as educational materials, field tests, and other assistance to resolve the residue problems on the farm before the animals are sent to market. When these efforts do not produce the desired results, the Agency implements intensive in-plant testing programs to detect the residues in the meat at slaughter and takes corresponding regulatory action against the offending producers.

Tests for Antibiotic Residues

FSIS currently uses a variety of tests for detecting antibiotic residues in meat; among these are field, in-plant, and laboratory screen tests, bioassays, immunoassays, and related biochemical techniques.

Field, In-Plant, and Laboratory Tests

FSIS has developed a series of overnight, inexpensive, easy to perform swab bioassay tests for screening tissues, body fluids, or feed extracts for antibiotic residues. The swab tests are used on the farm, in the slaughter plant, or in the laboratory for their designated purpose. Swab test results indicate whether antimicrobial activity is present in the sample at or above allowable levels or absent. Further testing with more sophisticated tests is required to identify and quantify the antibiotics producing the antimicrobial activity. These are usually done in a laboratory as required.

Basically, all swab tests are performed in the same manner. The analyst (farmer, veterinarian, laboratory scientist, or any other user) saturates a cotton tipped swab with sample tissue fluids, serum, urine, or feed extract. He then firmly places the saturated cotton swab on the surface of the appropriate growth medium previously surface streaked with the working dilution of the appropriate susceptible test organism. The test is then incubated at the proper temperature overnight and observed the next day for antimicrobial activity. If there is a zone of inhibition (no growth of the test organism) around the sample swab, the test is positive; no inhibition indicates that antimicrobials are absent or below detectable levels in the sample tested.

There are currently five swab tests in use:

- Live Animal Swab Test (LAST)
- Residue Avoidance Feed Test (RAFT)
- Swab Test on Premises (STOP)
- Calve Antibiotic/Sulfonamide Test (CAST)
- STOP II

LAST is used by farmers, veterinarians, and other interested parties to screen urine from cull dairy cows for antibiotic residues before marketing. If the LAST test is positive, the animal is retained for several days and retested before sale. A negative LAST test allows the farmer to market his cull cow with a high degree of confidence that the edible meat, liver, kidney, etc., at slaughter will be antibiotic residue free or below established tolerances.

RAFT allows feed mill operators, farmers, etc., to test feed or feed constituents for antimicrobial activity. A feed containing an antibiotic added intentionally (medicated feed) or unintentionally (contaminated feed) and detectable by RAFT will result in a positive RAFT test.

STOP is used by Federal Meat inspection personnel in-plant to check tissues from slaughtered animals for antibiotic residues.

Edible tissues from STOP-positive animals are retained until tested further by FSIS laboratories. If the laboratory report indicates antibiotic at or above tolerance levels, the viscera and/or the carcass are condemned. If antibiotic levels are below tolerance levels upon laboratory testing, the tissues are released into the food supply. In-plant STOP-negative animals are released without delay into the food chain. STOP may be used to test all food animals and poultry for antibiotic residues. Since STOP began in 1979, the incidence of antibiotic residues in the bovine meat supply has been reduced to approximately one percent.

CAST allows FSIS meat inspectors to test young veal calves at slaughter for antibiotic and sulfonamide residues. This category of veal animal has a lengthy past history of antibiotic misuse at slaughter. A positive CAST finding results in the animal's condemnation or requires further testing at an FSIS laboratory. A CAST-negative animal is released into the food chain without delay. The FSIS CAST program, started in June 1985, has been successful in reducing the incidence of antibiotics and sulfonamides in the veal supply.

STOP II currently is used exclusively by FSIS laboratories to screen import and domestic monitoring samples for tylosin, novobiocin, virginiamycin, and lincomycin. This test detects these compounds at or above established tolerance levels. Positive findings indicate that these drugs may be present and were not properly withdrawn before the animals was sold for slaughter.

Other tests used by FSIS to detect, identify, and/or quantify antibiotic residues in meat are primarily designed for laboratory use.

The conventional bioassays based on methodology developed by FDA and expanded by FSIS use four extractant buffers, five test organisms, five growth media, two incubation temperatures, and penicillinase to detect, identify, and/or quantify antibiotics such as the penicillins, streptomycins, tetracyclines, neomycins, erythromycin, tylosin, etc. Bioassay laboratory results are used by FSIS to take regulatory action and by FDA to prosecute farmers with histories of improperly withdrawing antibiotics before marketing their herds or flocks.

Certain drugs such as chloramphenicol require additional tests for their detection and quantification in meat tissues. The Competitive Enzyme Labeled Immunoassay for Chloramphenicol (CELIA) was developed and is used by FSIS laboratories to detect and quantify this drug in the meat supply; chloramphenicol is not approved for use in food animals. CELIA detects 5 ppb chloramphenicol in tissue extracts.

The antibiotic identification capabilities of FSIS laboratories have rapidly expanded during the past year. Commercially-produced ELISA-type immunoassays, such as the E-Z Screen, are being rapidly adapted by FSIS laboratories for use in testing meat extracts and body fluids for various antibiotics. These tests are relatively inexpensive, specific, sensitive to appropriate levels, and provide results on the same day. Within the next several years, FSIS laboratories will be able to screen for and confirm the presence of at least 22 different antibiotics.

Biochemical sophisticated separation techniques are also used when necessary to confirm and quantify immunoassay test results.

FSIS laboratories also use chemical techniques and instrumentation to identify select antibiotic residues. The tetracyclines of interest are identified by thin layer chromatography. Sulfonamides are detected and quantified by fluorescence thin lay chromatography and confirmed by gas chromatography/mass spectrometry. Amoxicillin and gentamycin are identified and/or quantified by high pressure liquid chromatography. Similar techniques are used to identify ionophores and other antimicrobials of interest.

In conclusion, FSIS is making a determined effort to reduce antibiotic and other man-incurred residues in the meat supply. The Agency is providing resources such as educational materials and inexpensive screen tests to industry for preventing antimicrobial residues in meat animals and poultry before marketing. Screen tests such as STOP and LAST are used in-plant by inspectors to check meat and poultry at slaughter. Additional in-plant screen tests are planned for introduction soon. Laboratory capabilities are also being rapidly expanded by improving the bioassays and by introducing rapid, sensitive, inexpensive ELISA-type immunoassays. Sophisticated biochemical/physical techniques are also in-place or under active evaluation.

RECEIVED May 2, 1986

13

Microbiological Assay Procedures for Antibiotic Residues

Stanley E. Katz

Department of Biochemistry and Microbiology, Rutgers University—The State University of New Jersey, New Brunswick, NJ 08903

>The classical microbial assay approaches to measuring antibiotic residues, diffusion, turbidimetric and acid production were described and the advantages and limitations reviewed. Other systems so discussed and reviewed were the affinity or receptor methods and the immunological approach using ELISA or EMIT assay techniques. The classical systems, in general, could measure antibiotic residues at the fractional ppm to the ppb levels. The potentials of the receptor and immunological assay system were discussed.

The appearance of antibiotic residues in food products of animal origin are for the most part the result of improper and careless usage, from deliberate and intentional misusage, from the improper formulation of animal feeding materials and from the ignoring of proper withdrawal times. The paths of misuse of antibiotics in animal agriculture can be as varied as the imagination of man can devise; all however, are based upon economic needs or perceived needs to prevent disease and/or to treat recalcitrant infections.

The analysis for antibiotic residues in edible animal tissue, eggs, milk, traditionally, has been performed using microbiological assay techniques. Primarily, these assay procedures were inhibition assays utilizing the agar diffusion systems (1). Microbiological assay procedures measure active species, i.e., those that can inhibit the growth of microorganisms. Metabolic products that are not inhibitory, are not measured; conjugated antibiotics, typically Phase II metabolites, usually will not be detected. Detection of such metabolic products requires hydrolysis of the conjugate prior to the assay.

Overall, microbiological assay methods have been the most sensitive of all assay systems and the ability to measure residues in the ppb to ppm range is common and has been for over 20 years (1). However, most of the residue assay systems lack specificity and require confirmation by spectral systems for a proper identification of the individual antibiotic or the antibiotic family.

There are many advantages to the use of microbial assay

methods. With rare exception, these procedures are simple to perform, possess a fair degree of precision and accuracy for the species they measure and require simple equipment to perform. Unfortunately, microbial systems are usually slow labor-intensive and require overnight incubations and multiple platings and measurements to achieve the ± 25% to ± 35% precision at the ppm to ppb concentration.

There are several ways to subdivide the analytical systems encompassing the area defined as microbial assay procedures. These are:
  Diffusion Systems
    cylinder-plate
    well-plate
    pad-plate
  Turbidimetric Systems
  Competitive Receptor Assays
  Immunological Systems

Diffusion Systems

Diffusion systems are based upon the ability of the antibiotic to diffuse through agar and cause the inhibition of the sensitive assay strains. Since the substrate to be assayed is applied in a "point source," diffusion occurs radially. A circular zone of inhibition forms and the size of the zone is a function of the concentration. This function is expressed as a linear relationship between the size of the zone of inhibition and the logarithm of the concentration. By comparing the measurable zone with a standard response line, the concentration of the dilution can be determined and the potency of the sample may be calculated. For a complete discussion of the mechanics of diffusion, the formation of the zone edge, and the relationships between concentration and zone size, the reader should refer to Kavanagh's classic text (2).

The Cylinder-Plate Procedure. In this procedure the substance being assayed diffuses from cylinders placed upon a uniform thickness of seeded agar, filled or charged with a fixed volume of the analyte, or reference standards or a series of standard solutions. The petri dishes are incubated at a predetermined temperature and the zones of inhibition measured to the nearest 0.1 mm.

The Cup-Plate or Well Procedure. This procedure is similar to the cylinder-plate system except that wells are cut into the agar with cutters capable of cutting uniform, completely circular wells. As with the cylinder-plate assays, the wells are filled. Zones are measured after incubation and the concentration determined utilizing a comparison with a standard response line.

The Pad-Plate Procedure. The pad-plate approach utilizes filter paper discs saturated with solution of the analyte as the reservoir. In all other respects, the system is identical to the other diffusion systems.

The advantages of the diffusion system are: (i) variations are adaptable to provide reasonably sensitive assays, (ii) the approach is adaptable to assay most if not all antibiotics, and (iii) the analyte solution need not be sterile or treated specially. The disadvantages are: (i) filling cylinder or wells or saturating and placing pads on agar pads is labor intensive, slow and tedious, (ii) most assays require overnight incubation and hence any assay covers a two-day period, and (iii) the pad-plate variation is the least sensitive usually capable of measuring µg/mL quantities; in comparison, the cylinder or well variation can measure ng/mL levels, suspended materials interfere in the cylinder-plate system by plugging the bottoms of the cylinder and limiting diffusion; in contrast the well system is unaffected since the analyte solution diffuses only horizontally rather than vertically and horizontally.

Several factors affect the diffusion assay and must be controlled carefully. The depth of the agar in the cylinder-plate system must be minimal, as thin as possible and as uniform as possible to maximize diffusion of the analyte.

The temperature of incubators must be uniform throughout and should not vary more than ± 0.2°C. The vegetative assay organism must be sensitive to the analyte, be stable (resistant to spontaneous change), be in the logarithmic growth phase (for uniformity of response), and be easily cultured, maintained and standardized. Spores suspension have similar criteria except that the spores must be capable of germinating with reasonable synchrony.

Utilizing the diffusion assay systems, primarily the cylinder-plate procedure, the following limits of detection and measurement are realistic.

Table I. Detection and Measurement Levels of Antibiotic Residues in Products of Animal Origin Using Diffusion Assays

Antibiotic	Milk	Dairy Products	Animal Muscle	Eggs	References
	µgs or units/g or mL				
Penicillins	0.005-0.01	0.01-0.02	0.01-0.02	0.025-0.03	(1) (3-13)
Streptomycins	0.06-0.10	0.20-0.40	0.20-0.40	0.30-0.50	(1) (14) (15)
Chlortetracycline	0.005-0.10	0.02-0.03	0.02-0.03	0.02-0.04	(1)(16-20)
Oxytetracycline	0.025-0.03	0.08-0.10	0.08-0.10	0.08-0.10	(1) (21-22)
Chloramphenicol	0.025-0.05	-	0.10-0.20	0.025-0.05	(1) (23)
Neomycin	0.05-0.10	-	0.25-0.50	0.20-0.30	(1) (24-25)
Erythromycin	0.025-0.05	0.10-0.20	0.10-0.20	0.10-0.20	(1) (26-27)

Some other antibiotics commonly used in animal production such as the bacitracins, bambermycins and virginiamycins as well as the streptomycins are poorly absorbed from the intestinal tract and residues usually do not occur from feeding. Chloramphenicol is used illegally in the United States in many species; it is used legally in Europe, Canada and other parts of the world.

The maximum sensitivity (the lower limit of detection and measurement) that can be achieved for any diffusion procedure is a function of the response of the test organism to the antibiotic being assayed. In order to increase the sensitivity of such procedures, an extraction system must be devised to concentrate the antibiotic. Solvent extraction and concentration, and subsequent partitioning into a suitable buffer has not achieved any large degree of success simply because of complications from co-extraction of interferences. Use of column concentration/clean-up techniques also has not been exploited since there appears to be little advantage to it, at present.

Interferences have been handled, traditionally, by the use of a matrix compensation response curve. Basically, the system is a series of standard additions to samples of a matrix and the use of these supplementations as the standards in a response curve. Thus, the recoveries of antibiotics, affected positively or negatively, can be corrected for matrix effects over a wide range of concentrations. Absolute recoveries are, of course, determined against standards in buffer.

Extractions traditionally have been performed using buffers (1); the same used to obtain the maximum response in standard curves. Unfortunately this has been a major failing of the plate diffusion assay systems. It is rare that the pH can be adjusted to the optimum necessary for greatest response simply by blending a matrix with buffer. As much as a 30 to 40% loss of activity can occur by not adjusting the pH properly; analysis for residues of the streptomycins and erythromycin, for example, can yield results 20% lower by having the pH of the analyte 0.2 units below 8.0; if the pH is 0.5 units below 8.0, the loss of potency approaches 50% (14-15).

The conventional assay systems (1) include dilutions of 1:2 to 1:5, as part of the extraction. Hence, the levels of detection are limited. The use of minimum amounts of extractant coupled with the physical removal of solids can improve the limits of detection and measurement.

Again, it is important to reiterate one important fact, only free antibiotic is measured. Bound residues are rarely measured directly using these assays. Another problem with all such assays is the supplementation system. The assumption that the simple addition of drug to a matrix followed by analysis was reflective of the problems of assaying for antibiotic residues is simplistic and does not address the overall problem of assaying for antibiotic residues.

Turbidimetric Systems

The methodology is based upon the relationship between the increasing concentrations of an antibiotic and the resulting inhibition of the growth of a microorganism as measured by the development of turbidity. The presence of increasing amounts of antibiotic in the assay medium result in an increasing inhibition of growth. By comparing the response of the assay organism exposed to an unknown quantity of antibiotic with the response found from known concentrations, the potency of the antibiotic in the sample can be determined (absorbance vs concentration). The procedure requires that the standards and the samples be assayed under exactly the same conditions. The most general method utilized is based upon the growth rate. This involves a short (usually 3-4 h) incubation period after which the incubation is terminated and the absorbance (turbidity) measured in a suitable spectrophotometer, using a flow-through cell system. Required for this assay are medium control, uniform test organism seeding, incubation temperature control, and a quenching system to cause the cessation of growth (2).

This approach has certain advantages over the diffusion system; it is more sensitive to low concentrations and the assay is rapid. However, the limitations precluded this approach from widespread application. Extracts of tissue or body fluids are often turbid or have interfering colors and can cause errors. Solvents can interfere much more in the turbidimetric systems than in diffusion systems. Surprisingly, sterility is not a significant problem unless the samples contain very large numbers of organisms. If one inoculates the assay medium to yield a density of 1×10^5 organisms/mL, in 4 h assuming no lag phase; the organism concentration would be 4×10^8 organisms/mL (assuming no inhibitory material and an organism generation time of 20 min). At 10^5 organisms/mL there is minimal measurable turbidity. Only if a rapid growing organism is present in large numbers in the sample extract would an interference be noted.

Competitive Receptor Assays

This assay, commonly referred to as the Charm Test, is based upon the affinity of antibiotics for specific sites on the cell wall of microorganisms and the irreversible binding of the antibiotic to these sites. By adding ^{14}C-labelled or ^{3}H-labelled antibiotic to a sample of milk, urine or the aqueous extract of tissues together followed by microbial binding sites and measuring the quantity of the labelled antibiotic that binds to the microbial sites, the antibiotic residue can be measured.

The competition for receptor sites prevents the radiolabelled antibiotic from binding. Thus the more radiolabelled antibiotic bound, the less antibiotic in the sample.

The Charm Test was initially applied to the analysis of β-lactam residues in milk although its application to the analysis of body, fluids, meat extracts, and fermentation broths was indicated. There appears to be no rationale why this basic procedure cannot be applied to all types of matrices (water, soil, animal feeds, premixes).

The primary application of the procedure is the determination of the presence or absence of β-lactam (7) residues in milk and secondarily to measure the levels quantitatively. The receptor assay system has now been expanded to qualitatively detect residues of tetracycline, erythromycin, streptomycin, chloramphenicol, novobiocin, and sulfamethazine in milk, serum and urine (Table II) (30).

Basically the procedure to detect β-lactam residues in milk is remarkably simple. A 5 mL sample of milk is used. To this is added the ^{14}C-labelled β-lactam and the bacterial receptor sites. The mixture is incubated for 4 min at 85°C to complete the competition for receptor sites and centrifuged. The supernatant is discarded, the pellet is washed gently so as not to disturb the pellet. The pellet is resuspended in water and scintillation fluid is added. For quantitative work, the sample is counted for 5 min, for screening purposes 1 min.

The labelled antibiotics contain either a ^{3}H- or ^{14}C-label.

An entire antibiotic screen can be carried out using 4 samples with the assay time being 15 min to 1 h depending upon whether the qualitative or quantitative mode is desired.

Table II. Limits of Detection and Measurement of Antibiotics

Antibiotic Family	Milk	Serum	Urine
		μgs or units/mL	
Penicillins	0.0025	0.0025	0.0025
Tetracyclines	0.25	0.25	--
Macrolides	0.05	0.05	0.05
Aminoglycosides	0.025	0.10	0.10
Chloramphenicol	0.020	0.50	--
Sulfonamides	0.025	0.25	0.25
Novobiocin	0.010	--	--

From these data the potential of the receptor assay is evident. Comparison with the microbial diffusion assay system, Table I, indicates that the levels of detection and measurement are reasonably similar. The receptor assay has the added virtue of allowing for the completion by the analysis within an hour, generally, rather than several hours or the next day.

Miscellaneous Assays for Residues of Antibiotics in Milk

In conjunction with the discussion of the receptor assay system, it is logical to discuss the variations of the plate assay systems and/or growth systems using colorimetric indicators of inhibition of metabolism or growth.

Disc Assay - This is the simplist of the procedures and involves the placing of a standard 1/2" disc saturated with milk onto the surface of B. stearothermophilus seeded agar plate and co-incubating with suitable control discs at 55° or 64°C until well-defined zones of inhibition are obtained, usually 3-4 h. Confirmation using penicillinase-treated milk is required. Zones 14.0 mm are positive. The lower limit of detection is 0.008 units penicillin/mL. This type of assay is simple, reasonably rapid and reasonably sensitive. Quantitation is possible by using graded concentrations of penicillin in the control milk. The technique is limited, however, to β-lactam antibiotics, primarily penicillin (8).

A variation of the disc assay is the quantitative estimate using a central point. Each petri dish contains three reference discs which contain 0.016 units penicillin/mL and three discs saturated with the unknown milk. A penicillinase disc is placed in the center of each plate to help confirm the presence of penicillin. Three plates are used for each milk sample; B. stearothermophilus is the assay organism. After incubation for 2-4 h, zones are measured and compared to the diameters of the reference concentration. Validity of the difference between zone size of the reference and sample is determined statistically. This procedure is less sensitive and attempts to set the qualitative presence of β-lactams at 0.016 units/mL rather than at lower levels (3).

Colorimetric Assay for β-Lactams

The system discussed, commercially known as the Delvotest (9-11), utilizes a strain of B. stearothermophilus which grows at a very rapid rate and produces acid from the nutrients in the medium in the absence of inhibitory substances. When inhibitory substances such as the β-lactam antibiotics are present, acid production is inhibited. By incorporating bromcresol purple in the medium, it is easy to observe acid production, a change from purple to yellow. Incubation is performed at 65°C for approximately 3 h.

Table III shows the actual combination of colors that can be obtained and their interpretation.

Table III. Interpretation of Delvotest Results

Sample Color	Heated Confirm	Penicillinase Treated	Interpretation
Yellow	--	--	-
Purple or Purple Yellow	Yellow	Yellow	+
Purple	Purple	Purple	-
Purple/Yellow	Purple/Yellow	Purple/Yellow	-
Purple	Purple	Yellow	+

The levels of detection are quite good and are shown for a number of dairy products in Table IV.

Table IV. Limits of Detection of β-Lactams in Milk Using the Delvotest System

Milk Type	Units Penicillin/mL
Raw	0.004-0.005
Skim	0.006
Low fat 1-2%	0.004-0.005
Homogenized	0.004-0.006
Half and Half	0.007

Other miscellaneous assays for penicillin or other β-lactams in milk is the Penzyme Test which uses cell wall enzymes inhibited by β-lactam drugs in a kinetic assay. This test system is purported to be able to detect 0.005 units penicillin/mL and requires approximately 30 min to complete. It, like many other assays, detects β-lactam antibiotics only.

Application of Delvotest or the disc assay systems to detecting other antibiotics in milk has not been successful. Only the receptor assay system appears to be versatile and potentially applicable to determine the presence of different antibiotic residues in different matrices.

Immunological Systems

Microbiologically based assay systems invariably measure the active antibiotic(s) or forms of the antibiotic that can be inhibitory to microorganisms. Immunological assays can measure both the active antibiotic as well as microbiologically inactive species.

Immunological assays measure those moieties that can cause an antigenic response. For the most part, immunological assays should not be interfered with by antibiotics from the other antibiotic families, the specificity of the antibodies being vaguely similar to the specificity of enzyme systems.

The basic principle governing immunoassays for antibiotics is indicated in the following reaction:

$$Ag + Ab \rightleftharpoons Ag:Ab$$
$$\text{Antigen} \quad \text{Antibody} \quad \text{Antigen:Antibody Complex}$$

This reaction is an equilibrium reaction and will continue until the concentration of antigen in both the free and complexed form becomes a constant (30).

Applications of the immunological systems are limited by the ability to develop suitable antibodies. Most antibiotics are relatively small molecules having molecular weights under 500. Hence these molecules must be complexed with some carrier protein to create a molecule that can evoke the immune response and the development of antibodies.

An antibody is produced when the antigen carrying a number of antigenic determinants is introduced into an animal's body. Lines of B cells mature into plasma cells and each produces an immunoglobulin molecule that fits a single determinant or a segment of the determinant. In a conventional sense, antibodies are polyclonal proteins because they can be directed against several other components rather than against the antigen alone. Separation of the different antibodies in a polyclonal mixture is extremely difficult if not impossible. In contrast, monoclonal antibodies are directed against a specific antigen or a specific segment of the antigenic molecule.

Kohler and Milstein (31) revolutionized immunology by demonstrating that antibody producing cells (spleen cells) when fused with malignant mouse myeloma cells produced hybrid cell lines whose cells produced only a single antibody. These hybrid cells, known as hybridomas, were essentially immortal meaning that they could be grown in cell culture. A complete discussion of the production of antibody by hybridoma is given by Goding (32).

Immunological Techniques for Analyzing Antibiotics

Over the last 8-10 years, monoclonal as well as conventional antibody techniques have gained popularity for the analysis of hormones, various drugs, proteins, bacteria, viruses and parasites. Application of immunological systems for the analysis of drug and antibiotic residues has lagged because of the general lack of familiarity with the principles of immunology, the difficulties in producing stable reagents, and the difficulties in developing methods using the crude material initially available.

Agglutination. The agglutination assay or the passive hemagglutination inhibition assay is based upon the least amount of soluble antigen necessary to inhibit agglutination or the clumping of cells that occurs following the union of antigen and antibody.

Analytically this is the amount of antigen in the last tube of a dilution series that will give a wide ring agglutination pattern. Tubes containing less antigen than this tube allow agglutination to occur. It is quite common to use a two-fold dilution sequence - obviously the greater the interval between concentration, the greater the inaccuracy. The converse is also evident, the narrower the range, the greater the accuracy.

Application of this technique is very limited for assaying antibiotic residues. Steiner (33) developed such a model system utilizing gentamicin as the pilot antibiotic in matrices such as urine, blood serum, milk and animal feeds. The procedure was relatively simple. A measured volume of a gentamicin-treated red cell suspension was added to the previously mentioned gentamicin supplemented matrices. A fixed volume of gentamicin antibody was added and the mixture incubated at room temperature for 30 to 60 min. The hemagglutination reactions were observed and the concentration of antibiotic determined. The limits of this system for gentamicin were 0.4 ppm for chicken serum, burnine, 1.9 ug/mL for milk and 20 g/ton for feeds. Although these levels are not especially sensitive, the hemagglutination offers two distinct advantages, speed of analysis and specificity. The total assay usually can be completed within 2 h with no observable interferences from other antibiotics.

Radioimmunoassay. Radioimmunoassay (RIA) was first described by Berson and Yalow (34) and Luft and Yalow (35). The assay is based upon the competition for an antibody between a radiolabelled antigen and its unlabelled counterpart. The greater the amount of unlabelled antigen in the test sample, the less radiolabelled antigen bound. The concentration of antigen in a test sample can be determined from comparisons with standard curves.

The primary application of RIA for antibiotics has been in the medical area, and primarily for antibiotics not used in agriculture. Assays have been developed for gentamicin tobramycin, sisomicin, netilmicin and for hygromycin B, an antibiotic used primarily in agriculture (36-37, 22-24). Gentamycin could be measured as low as 80 pg, tobramycin 280 pg, netilmicin 300 pg mL.

The RIA has definite advantages, small samples, sizes, speed, accuracy, precision, specificity. There are significant disadvantages also. The labelled reactant is unstable (^{125}I) and costs are relatively high. The great sensitivity requires considerable dilutions; antibody-bound fractions must be separate from free fractions in order to obtain accurate counts.

In a sense, the receptor assay system is a RIA-type technique that has been applied to antibiotic residue analysis.

Nonisotopic Immunoassays. Nonisotopic immunoassays differ from the isotopic assays only in the type of label used, the end-point measurement, and the separation of bound and free fractions (41-43).

Fluoroimmunoassays. This assay requires the drug being assayed to be labelled with umbelliferyl-β-D-galactoside. The enzyme β-galactosidase is added and the fluorescent products are released from the labelled antibiotic. The antibody in the bound fraction inhibits the enzymatic hydrolysis. The differential in fluorescence is proportional to the antibiotic concentration. This technique could offer an excellent approach if endogenous fluorophores can be removed or minimized.

Enzyme Multiplied Immunoassay Technique (EMIT). This technique employs enzyme-labelled antibiotics which react analogously to the fluroimmunoassay in that a reduction of enzyme activity is attributed to antibody binding. Higher concentrations of unlabelled drug in the sample result in less enzyme-labelled drug bound to the antibody.

To perform the EMIT assay is rather simple and straightforward:
The sample is added to a plastic tube.
  [Substrate-antibody reagents could be
    β-NAD (β-nicotinamidoadenine dinucleotide and 1-malic acid)
    β-NAD and glucose-6-phosphate]
The enzyme reagent is added.
  malic dehydrogenase
  glucose-6-dehydrogenase
The reaction is stopped after 10 min with sodium borate.
Measure the intensity of the resulting color.

The range of antibiotic that can be measured is usually 0.01 to 1.00 ug antibiotic/mL and has been used for gentamicin, carbenicillin, ticarcillin and amikacin (44-46). The use of the EMIT system, to-date, has been in the clinical area and unrelated to measuring residues of antibiotics. The procedure has potential for residue analysis if interferences by non-specific factors can be overcome.

Enzyme-Linked Immunosorbent Assays (ELISA). Three methods are commonly used: direct competition, double antibody sandwich and antibody inhibition.

Direct competition. The solid phase (a microtiter plate) is coated with an antibody specific for the antigen being assayed. The sample and enzyme-labelled antigen (antibiotic) are added. There is a competition for the antibody between the labelled and unlabelled antigen (antibiotic). Substrate is added and the color produced by the enzymatic hydrolyse is inversely proportioned to the concentration of antigen in the sample (48).

Double-antibody sandwich. Antibody is coated on or adsorbed to the plastic plate. The sample to be assayed containing the antigen (antibiotic) is added followed by a second antibody that is conjugated to the enzyme (horseradish peroxidase, alkaline phosphatase, or β-galactosidase). The substrate is added and the intensity of the color produced is directly proportional to the antigen in the test sample.

Antibody inhibition. Antibody is preincubated with the sample being assayed. If any antigen is present in the sample it will bind with antibody. When the assay mixture is added to a microtiter plate coated with antigen, there is a decrease in the intensity of the color produced.

The aforementioned procedures (techniques) have significant potential and as assay problems are worked out could provide rapid, sensitive, specific and precise methods for the analysis of low levels of antibiotics in food and feed products.

Acknowledgments

New Jersey Agricultural Experiment Station Publication Number F-01112-01-86 supported by State and U. S. Hatch Act Funds.

Literature Cited

1. Kramer, J.; Carter, G. G.; Arret, B.; Wilner, J.; Wright, W. W.; Kirshbaum, A. Methods, Reports, and Protocols. Food and Drug Administration, Washington, D.C., 1968.
2. Kavanagh, F. "Analytical Microbiology"; Academic: New York, 1971; Vol. II.
3. Ginn, R. E.; Case, R. A.; Packard, V. S.; Tatini, S. R. J. Assoc. Off. Anal. Chem. 1982, 1407-12.
4. Katz, S. E.; Fassbender, C. A.; Hackett, A. J.; Mitchell, R. G. J. Assoc. Off. Anal. Chem. 1974, 57, 819-22.
5. Katz, S. E.; Fassbender, C. A. J. Assoc. Off. Anal. Chem. 1978, 61, 918-22.
6. Kelley, W. N. J. Assoc. Off. Anal. Chem. 1982, 65, 1193-1207.
7. Messer, J. W.; Leslie, J. E.; Houghtby, G. A.; Peeler, J. T.; Barnett, J. E. J. Assoc. Off. Anal. Chem. 1982, 65, 1208-14.
8. Ouderkirk, L. A. J. Assoc. Off. Anal. Chem. 1979, 62, 985-88.
9. Packard, V. S.; Tatini, S.; Ginn, R. E. J. Milk Food Technol. 1975, 38, 601-03.
10. Van Os, J. L.; Beukers, R. J. Food Protection. 1980, 43, 510-11.
11. Van Os, J. L.; Lameris, S. A.; Doodeward, T.; Oostendorp, J. G. Netherlands Milk Dairy J. 1975, 29, 16-34.
12. Katz, S. E.; Fassbender, C. A.; Dinnerstein, P. S.; Dowling, Jr., J. J. J. Assoc. Off. Anal. Chem. 1974, 57, 522-26.
13. Katz, S. E.; Fassbender, C. A.; DePaolis, A. M.; Rosen, J. D. J. Assoc. Off. Anal. Chem. 1978, 61, 564-68.
14. Inglis, J. M.; Katz, S. E. J. Assoc. Off. Anal. Chem. 1978, 61, 1098-1102.
15. Inglis, J. M.; Katz, S. E. Appl. Environ. Microbiol. 1978, 35, 517-20.
16. Katz, S. E.; Fassbender, C. A. J. Assoc. Off. Anal. Chem. 1970, 53, 968-72.
17. Katz, S. E.; Fassbender, C. A. J. Agr. Food Chem. 1970, 18, 1164-67.
18. Katz, S. E.; Fassbender, C. A.; Dorfman, D. Bull. Environ. Contam. Toxicol. 1971, 6, 110-16.
19. Katz, S. E.; Fassbender, C. A.; Dowling, J. J. J. Assoc. Off. Anal. Chem. 1972, 55, 123-33.
20. Katz, S. E.; Fassbender, C. A.; Dorfman, D.; Dowling, Jr., J. J. J. Assoc. Off. Anal. Chem. 1972, 55, 134-38.
21. Katz, S. E.; Fassbender, C. A. Bull. Environ. Contam. Toxicol. 1972, 7, 229-36.
22. Katz, S. E.; Fassbender, C. A.; Dowling, Jr., J. J. J. Assoc. Off. Anal. Chem. 1973, 56, 77-81.
23. Singer, C. J.; Katz, S. E. J. Assoc. Off. Anal. Chem. 1985, 1037-41.
24. Katz, S. E.; Levine, P. R. J. Assoc. Off. Anal. Chem. 1978, 61, 1103-06.

25. Levine, P. R. Ph.D. Thesis, Rutgers University, New Brunswick, N. J., 1980.
26. Harpster, C. P.; Katz, S. E. J. Assoc. Off. Anal. Chem. 1980, 63, 1144-48.
26a. Harpster, C. A. Ph.D. Thesis, Rutgers University, New Brunswick, N. J., 1979.
27. Charm, S. E. U.S. Patents 5 238 521; 4 239 745; 4 239 852, 1980.
28. Charm, S. E. Cultured Dairy Products J. 1979, 14, 24-26.
29. Charm, S. E.; Chi, R. K. J. Assoc. Off. Anal. Chem. 1982, 65, 1186-92.
30. Sell, S. "Immunology, Immunopathology and Immunity"; Harper and Row: Hagerstown, 1980; 3rd Ed.
31. Kohler, G.; Milstein, C. Nature. 1975, 256, 495-97.
32. Goding, J. W. J. Immunol. Meth. 1980, 39, 285-308.
33. Steiner, S. J. Ph.D. Thesis, Rutgers University, New Brunswick, N. J., 1981.
34. Berson, S. A.; Yalow, R. S. In "Radioimmunoassay: A Status Report in Immunology"; Good, R. A.; Fisher, D. W., Eds.; Sinauer: Stanford, 1971.
35. Luft, R.; Yallow, R. S. "Radioimmunoassay Methodology and Applications in Physiology and in Clinical Studies"; George Thieme Verlag: Stuttgard, 1974.
36. Broughton, A.; Strong, J. E.; Pickering, L. K.; Bodey, G. P. Antimicrob. Agents Chemother. 1976, 10, 652-56.
37. Lewis, J. E.; Nelson, J. C.; Elder, H. A. Nature New Biol. 1972, 239, 214-16.
38. Watson, R. A. A.; Wenk, M. In "Current Chemotherapy"; Siegenthaler, W.; Lathy, R., Eds.; American Society for Microbiology: Washington, D.C., 1978; Vol. 2.
39. Watson, R. A. A.; Shaw, E. J.; Edwards, G. R. W. In "Chemotherapy"; Williams, J. D.; Goeddes, A. M., Eds.; Plenum: New York, 1976; Vol. 2.
40. Foglesong, M. A.; LeFeber, D. S. J. Assoc. Off. Anal. Chem. 1982, 65, 48-51.
41. Shaw, E. J.; Watson, R. A. A.; Landon, J.; Smith, D. S. J. Clin. Pathol. 1977, 30, 526-31.
42. Shaw, E. J.; Watson, R. A. A.; Smith, D. A. Clin. Chem. 1979, 25, 322-24.
43. Bund, J.; Wong, R. C.; Feeney, J. E.; Carrico, R. J.; Boguslaski, R. C. Clin. Chem. 1977, 23, 1402-08.
44. O'Leary, T. D.; Ratcliff, R. M.; Geary, T. D. Antimicrob. Agents Chemother. 1980, 17, 776-78.
45. Erwin, J. R.; Bullock, W. E.; Nattall, C. E. Antimicrob. Agents Chemother. 1976, 9, 1004-11.
46. Hindler, J. Abstracts, Annual American Society for Microbiology Meeting, 1983.
47. Voller, A.; Bidwell, D. E.; Bartlett, A. "The Enzyme-linked Immunosorbent Assay (ELISA), A Guide with Abstracts of Micro-Plate Applications"; Dynatech Publication, Nuffield Laboratories of Comparative Medicine; Zoological Soc. of London: Reagents Park.
48. Campbell, G. S.; Mageau, R. P.; Schwab, B.; Johnston, R. W. Antimicrob. Agents Chemother. 1984, 25, 205-11.

RECEIVED May 8, 1986

14

Physicochemical Methods for Identifying Antibiotic Residues in Foods

William A. Moats

Meat Science Research Laboratory, Agricultural Research Service, U.S. Department of Agriculture, Beltsville, MD 20705

> The physicochemical methods are needed for identification and quantitation of antibiotic residues in milk and tissues of animals. Methods successfully employed include high voltage electrophoresis with detection by bioautography and chromatographic procedures. Gas-liquid (GLC), thin-layer (TLC) and high performance liquid chromatography (HPLC) have all been used for residue analysis. A number of chromatographic methods have been described for chloramphenicol and the sulfonamides using all three chromatographic modes. Less work has been reported with residues of other antibiotics. Satisfactory physicochemical confirmatory tests are not available for some compounds.

The work on residue monitoring has been divided into microbiological methods covered in the preceding chapter and physicochemical methods which is the topic of this chapter. The division between the two approaches is somewhat arbitrary since many methods include elements of both approaches. Physicochemical methods are commonly used for identification and/or quantitation of residues detected by various types of screening methods, although they can be used for direct testing for residues. Successful methods mainly employ either high voltage electrophoresis or chromatography for separation of compounds and I will discuss application of these two approaches to residues in food substrates. For the present discussion, sulfonamides are also included, since they are used in a similar manner to antibiotics.

Electrophoresis

High voltage electrophoresis (HVE) in agar gel with detection by bioautography has been used with considerable success in some laboratories for identification of residues (1-6). This procedure has the advantage that all antibiotic substances detectable by bioautography can be classified on the basis of electrophoretic mobility. Further testing may be required for quantification and to distinguish compounds with similar electrophoretic mobilities, especially if only one buffer is used (7,8). Natural microbial inhibitors found in some animal tissues form a streak unlike any antibiotic compound. Smither et al (9) examined 5442 UK-produced meat samples using the four plate test (FPT) of the European community. Of these, 34 were initially positive. However, electrophoresis demonstrated that only two of the positives were recognizable antibiotics. On retesting, 20 of the samples originally positive were negative and 12 samples were found to contain natural microbial inhibitors. Van Schothorst and Van Leusden (5) reported good agreement between electrophoresis and bioassays for confirmation of residues found in kidney. Engel et al (10) found that of residues detected in kidney and muscle by the European four-plate test (FPT), only 50% and 37%, respectively, could be confirmed by HVE. They concluded that HVE is less sensitive than the FPT.

Chromatographic Methods

Enough chromatographic methods for antibiotics have been described to warrant a book on the subject (11). These are, however, mainly for formulations and clinical applications and application to residue analysis has been rather limited. Residue analysis requires greater sensitivity and isolation from more complex substrates than is the case with other applications. However, considerable progress has been reported in recent years, especially with chloramphenicol and the sulfonamides. Thin layer chromatography (TLC), high performance liquid chromatography (HPLC), and gas liquid chromatography (GLC) have all been used. The applications of GLC for analysis of drug residues in tissues were recently reviewed by Petz (12). Chromatographic methods are frequently suitable for determination of residues of a number of compounds in a single procedure. They also have the potential to detect metabolites. Further confirmation by spectrophotometry and/or mass spectrometry is possible. A discussion of the application to specific antibiotic residues follows.

Sulfonamides

Rapid progress has been reported in the development of methods for sulfonamide residues in tissues, milk, and eggs since the subject was reviewed by Horwitz (13) in 1981. The colorimetric method of Tishler et al (14) has in the past been used to detect violative levels of sulfonamide residues in animal tissues. The lack of specificity and the variable background levels produced by this method have been discussed by Horwitz (13), Matusik et al (15), and Lloyd et al (16). Recently, a number of specific chromatographic methods have been described for determination of residues of a variety of sulfonamides. These are summarized in Table I and suggest that HPLC is emerging as the method of choice followed by GLC and TLC methods. The methods listed do not include a number described for blood and/or urine only.

The HPLC methods mainly use UV detectors, but one uses amperometric (18) and one uses fluorescent detection (25). Fluorescent detection after derivatization with fluorescamine is the method most commonly used for detection on TLC plates. Vilim (24) used TLC to

Table I. Chromatographic Methods for Determination of Sulfonamide Residues in Tissue, Milk, and Eggs

Method	Substrate	Compounds	Detection	Sensitivity (ppb)	Reference
HPLC	Chicken, tissue eggs	SFX, SMM[a/] SDM, SQX	UV	5	(17)
	Liver, kidney muscle	Several	Amperometric	10	(18)
	Chicken tissue	SQX	UV	10	(19)
	Chicken tissue	SMM, SDN, SQX	UV	10-30	(20)
	Swine liver	Glycopyranosyl SMZ	UV	10	(21)
	Chicken tissue, eggs	SQX	UV	10-30	(22)
	Beef tissue	SMZ	UV	100	(23)
	Pork tissue	SMZ	UV	50	(24)
	Chicken tissue, eggs	SMM, BDM, SQX	Fluorescamine Derivative	--	(25)
	Eggs, meat, milk	SMR, SDZ SDD, SMX, SQX	UV	100	(26)
	Swine tissue	SMZ	UV	50	(27)
	Swine tissue	5	UV	50	(28)
TLC	Pork liver	SMZ, STH	Colorimetric	100	(29)
	Liver, muscle	SMZ, SDM STH, SQX SBM	Fluorescamine Quantity	<100	(30, 31)
	Tissues	5	Fluorescamine	50	(32)
	Tissues	23	Fluorescamine	100	(33)
	Tissues	18	Fluorescamine	10	(34)
	Swine tissue	5	Fluorescamine	50	(35)

Table I. Chromatographic Methods for Determination of Sulfonamide Residues in Tissue, Milk, and Eggs (Continued)

Method	Substrate	Compounds	Detection	Sensitivity (ppb)	Reference
GLC	Cattle, swine tissues	SMZ	MS	100	(36)
	Tissues	SMZ	EC-MS	100	(15)
	Cattle, swine	7	EC	100	(37)
	Cattle, swine tissues	SDM	MS	100	(38)
	Swine tissue 14_C	SMZ and metabolites	MS	2-12	(39)
	Swine tissue	SMZ	MS	100	(40)
	Swine tissue	SMZ	MS	100	(41)
	Swine tissue	SMZ	MS	100	(42)
MS (Direct)	Swine liver	18	CID/MIKE	100	(43)

a/ Abbreviations: SMM - sulfomonomethoxine; SFX - sulfisoxazol; SDM - Sulfadimethoxine; SQX - sulfaquinoxaline; SMZ - sulfamethazine; TMP - trimethoprim; STH - sulfathiazole; SDZ - sulfadiazine; SMR - sulfamerazine; SDD - sulfadimidine (syn. for sulfamethazine); SBM - sulfabromomethazine; MS - mass spectrometry; EC - electron capture.

confirm HPLC results. A number of GLC methods have also been described, most of which use mass spectrometry (MS) for confirmation. Brumley et al (42) describe a method for identifying sulfonamide residues in extracts of swine liver by a procedure known as collision-induced dissociation/mass analyzed ion kinetic energy spectrometry (CID/MIKE). This method was applied to the determination of 18 compounds. Only a few methods (15,38) address the determination of metabolites. When tissue samples are allowed to stand (44) or are stored frozen (21), sulfonamides present are converted to the N^4-glucopyranosyl derivatives which can give confusing and misleading results.

Schlatterer and Weise (45) compared a microbiological inhibition test with TLC for detection of sulfonamides in kidneys and muscles of slaughtered animals. About 30% of kidney samples positive by the microbiological assay were negative by TLC. Conversely, 30% of muscle samples positive by TLC did not give a positive microbiological test.

Chloramphenicol

Methods for chloramphenicol were recently reviewed by Allen (46) and also by Milhaut (47). Chloramphenicol is widely used in Europe. In the United States, its use in food-producing animals is not permitted, but there is considerable evidence that it is used illegally (46,48). Most microbiological screening procedures are relatively insensitive to chloramphenicol and will detect only high levels of the compound (49). Metabolites such as the glucuronide do not inhibit microorganisms unless they are hydrolyzed (50).

Allen (46) summarized 24 methods employed for detection and quantitation of chloramphenicol residues in milk, eggs, and tissues. Of these, eight used GLC, nine used HPLC, six used TLC, and one used column chromatography in conjunction with a color test. Four methods used GC/MS for residue confirmation. A rapid, sensitive (0.1 ppb) GC method for chloramphenicol in milk was recently described (51). Although there is evidence that a significant part of chloramphenicol residues in tissues of treated animals is present as the glucuronide (50,52), only one method (52) used glucuronidase treatment prior to extractions of residues. Nouws (50) noted that chloramphenicol residues in kidneys were rapidly converted to the arylamine form post mortem and suggested testing residual urine after glucuronidase treatment to free chloramphenicol.

Tetracyclines

A number of methods have been described for determination of tetracycline (chlortetracycline, tetracycline, and oxytetracycline) residues in tissues of food-producing animals (53-62), fish (63), eggs (64), and honey (65,66). Most of these methods use reversed-phase HPLC for determination. However, one uses TLC with UV densitometry (63) and one uses GLC (58), and one uses a direct mass spectrometric method: CAD MIKE spectrometry (collisionally activated decomposition mass-analyzed ion kinetic spectrometry) for oxytetracycline in milk and meat (62). Several use solid-phase extraction in the cleanup procedure using XAD-2 resin (56,58) or C_{18} cartridges

(59-61,63,66). Nelis and DeLeenheer (67) described a method for determining doxycycline in human tissues.

A number of problems have been encountered in determination of tetracyclines. These include:

1. Poor reproducibility of chromatographic methods because of interactions with the silica support of bonded reversed-phase columns (54,56,68,69).
2. Difficulty in resolving oxytetracycline and tetracycline (56,57,69).
3. Poor recoveries, especially from tissue samples (54,59,63).
4. Losses during concentration of sample extracts by evaporation (57).

We have addressed these problems in our laboratory (53) and have developed an improved procedure for residues of chlortetracycline, oxytetracycline, and tetracycline in tissues which avoids these problems by:

1. Acid-acetonitrile extraction of residues.
2. Direct concentration by solid-phase extraction on the analytical column, eliminating the evaporation step.
3. Use of an all organic polymeric column or adding a silanol blocking agent, tetramethyl ammonium chloride to the mobile phase to eliminate silanol-tetracycline interactions. This resulted in a rapid simplified method which gave 80-100% recoveries of tetracyclines with good sensitivity and resolution.

B-lactam Antibiotics

Although many B-lactam antibiotics have been described, a relatively small number are used in food-producing animals and these are the only ones of concern as residues. Microbiological test procedures are ordinarily very sensitive to B-lactam antibiotics (49). Tolerances for these compounds are generally 0-.01 ppm except for penicillin G in cattle (.05 ppm) and cephapirin in edible tissue (0.1 ppm) and milk (.02 ppm) (70). Many chromatographic methods have been described for determination of these compounds in clinical applications, but these methods are not sufficiently sensitive for residue analysis. The summary of methods in Table II includes one GLC (71), five TLC (72-76), and five HPLC methods (77-81). Four of the TLC methods use detection by bioautography. Three HPLC methods have been described for milk (77-79) and two for tissue (80,81). The HPLC methods described by Moats (78,80) and by Munns et al (77) are satisfactory for any penicillin with a neutral side-chain and this may be true with the procedure of Terada, et al. (81). The procedure of Terada and Sakabe (79) is also satisfactory for the aminopenicillin, ampicillin. The method of Munns et al (77) can also be used to detect the corresponding penicilloic acid metabolites.

In a comparison with microbiological methods for penicillin in milk, Moats concluded that the TLC (75) and HPLC (78) methods described for milk were comparable in sensitivity for penicillin G and far more sensitive for cloxacillin. Other reported methods vary greatly in sensitivity. The two reported HPLC methods for

Table II. Chromatographic Methods for Detection of B-lactam Antibiotic Residues in Foods

Method	Substrate	Compounds	Extraction/cleanup	Detection	Sensitivity (ppb)	Reference
GLC						
	Milk	Ox, Clox, Diclox	CHCl₃ partitioning	ECD	10	(71)
TLC						
	Milk	PG, Clox, Ceph, Amp	none	Bioautography	1 PG; 3 Amp, Ceph; 20 Clox	(72)
	Muscle, kidney	PG, Amp	none	Bioautography	100	(73)
	Muscle	Amp	none	Bioautography	10	(74)
	Milk	PG, Clox	CH₃CN/partitioning	Colorimetric	4PG, Clox	(75)
	Milk	Amp, Ox, Clox	Organic solvents	Bioautography	1000 Clox 500 Ox 100 Amp	(76)

HPLC

Sample	Drugs	Cleanup	Detection	Sensitivity (ppb)	Ref.
Milk	8 with neutral side chains – also penicilloates	CH$_3$CN/partitioning	Fluorometric	20–50	(77)
Milk	PG, PV, Clox	CH$_3$CN/partitioning	UV 220 nm	5PG, PV, 2 Clox	(78)
Milk	PG, PV, Amp	Sep-pak C$_{18}$	UV	30	(79)
Tissue	PG, Clox	CH$_3$CN/partitioning	UV 220 nm	50PG, 20 Clox	(80)
Tissue	PG	Tungstic acid, sep-pak, alumina	UV	50	(81)

PG – penicillin G; PV – penicillin V; Clox – cloxacillin; Diclox – dicloxacillin; Ceph – Cephapirin; Ox – oxacillin, Amp – ampicillin, ECD – Electron capture detection

a/ Tolerances (U.S.): Edible tissue (cattle) – 0.05 ppm PG, 0.1 ppm Ceph; others – 0–0.01 ppm; milk – 0.02 ppm Ceph; others 0 (65).

penicillin G in tissues (80,81) are barely adequate to detect it at the tolerance of .05 ppm in beef tissue. It should not be assumed that microbiological methods are necessarily more sensitive for residues in tissues. Natural microbial inhibitors are frequently encountered in animal tissues (49,82) and detection of residues at <0.1 ppm becomes increasingly uncertain.

Penicillins form several major metabolites which are excreted in the urine (83,84). These metabolites are usually inactive microbiologically and they would not be detected by the usual microbiological tests. There are no analytical methods for these metabolites in tissues and, therefore, little is known as to their occurrence and persistence in tissues. There are no methods available for identifying residues of some commonly used B-lactam antibiotics including carbenicillin and ticarcillin. For cephapirin and ampicillin, except for one HPLC method for ampicillin in milk (79) only TLC procedures (72-74,76) with detection by bioautography are reported.

We compared our HPLC method for penicillin G with a microbiological test for residues in tissues of treated swine (82). The HPLC method frequently gave results several-fold higher than the microbiological test. The swine tissues frequently contained natural inhibitors which interfered with detection of penicillin at <0.1 ppm in tissues. It is commonly assumed that penicillins can be distinguished from natural inhibitors by treatment with penicillinase. However, tissues, especially kidneys, of control pigs with no history of exposure to B-lactam antibiotics contained inhibitors inactivated by penicillin. These inhibitors were carried through the cleanup used for penicillin G but they were not penicillin G by HPLC. The cleanup used is specific for organic acids and will only recover B-lactam antibiotics with neutral side-chains. At present, we do not know whether or not the inhibitor is in fact a B-lactam antibiotic. There is no reason to suppose it is. These results emphasize the need for specific confirmatory tests since considerable economic losses could result from misidentification of residues.

Macrolide Antibiotics

The application of chromatographic methods to analyze the residues of macrolide antibiotics has been very limited. Moats (85) listed four TLC and one HPLC method for tylosin and one TLC method for erythromycin. In a comparison of the HPLC and microbiological methods for incurred residues in swine, the HPLC method was more sensitive and usually gave higher results (86).

Ionophores

Weiss and MacDonald (87) recently reviewed methods for determination of ionophore antibiotics. Ionophores approved for use in animal agriculture in the U.S. are lasalocid, monensin, and salinomycin. An HPLC (88) and GLC-MS (89) procedure have been described for lasalocid. For other ionophores, TLC-bioautography is the preferred procedure because of lack of any useful UV absorbance. However, a few TLC colorimetric procedures have been described for monensin residues in tissues (90-92).

Aminoglycosides

Although a number of chromatographic methods have been reported for determinations of aminoglycoside antibiotics in blood serum and urine, the application of chromatographic methods to residue analysis has been very limited. Shaikh et al (93) recently described an HPLC method for neomycin in animal tissue, and Lachatre et al (94) described a method for nine aminoglycosides in plasma, urine, and renal cortex tissue. Both procedures use post column derivatization with σ-pthalaldehyde and fluorescence detection.

Summary and Conclusions

Although some European countries still accept the results of the four plate test as confirming the presence of antibiotic residues in samples (9), other work indicates that FPT test is not necessarily reliable. The occurrence of natural microbial inhibitors in tissues has frequently been noted (4,9,49,82). It has also been frequently observed that the results obtained by microbial and physicochemical procedures sometimes differ considerably (9,10,45,82,86). Results obtained in our laboratory suggest that even inactivation by penicillinase may not be totally specific for B-lactam antibiotics (82). The specificity of immunoassay procedures depends on the specificity of the antibody used in the test (95). Specific antisera are not widely available at present. Physicochemical procedures are therefore essential for identification and confirmation of suspect residues detected by microbiological tests.

The review of the literature demonstrates considerable progress in recent years, especially for sulfonamides and chloramphenicol. Specific methods are still lacking for many antibiotics. Recently, Thomas Dols of the U.S. Food and Drug Administration testified before a Congressional committee that methods are available for detecting residues of only 29% of the animal drugs for which tolerances have been set (96). Although not broken down, this figure certainly includes many antibiotic compounds. Physicochemical methods also have the potential to detect microbiologically inactive metabolites. However, progress in this area has been limited. There is evidence that a significant portion of sulfonamide and chloramphenicol residues are present as metabolites in tissue (21,39,44,46,50,52). It is also known that penicillins are partially converted to penicilloates and other metabolites before they are excreted in the urine (83,84). The occurrence of metabolites in tissue and milk is unknown. The penicillin metabolites are potentially as allergenic as the parent compounds (97). In biological materials, reversible binding of drugs to proteins can also occur and that can affect analytical results (98,99). Antibiotics or metabolites are bound covalently to proteins and persist for an extended period in tissues or blood (100,101, D. Berkowitz, personal comm.). The amount bound is insignificant from the standpoint of pharmacologic disposition of the antibiotic but is of possible concern because of its persistence. Covalently bound residues are not detected by the usual microbiological or chemical tests but might be detected by immunoassay. The significance of such bound residues is unknown.

There is clearly a need for a great deal more work to develop specific test methods for residues and to establish the reliability of proposed rapid test procedures. Of physicochemical methods, high voltage electrophoresis with bioautography is useful in classifying unknown residues. Although antibiotics are generally not very volatile, GLC with confirmation by mass spectrometry has been used to some extent, especially with sulfonamides and chloramphenicol. There are also reports of the direct use of mass spectrometry on sample extracts (43,62). HPLC is emerging as the method of choice with rapid development in equipment, column packings, and detectors. Direct injection of blood serum (102) or sample extracts with little or no cleanup (53) is possible, which makes HPLC procedures comparable in speed with other rapid tests. With increased use of solid-phase absorption in cleanup, automation of procedures is feasible. TLC is also a useful and inexpensive technique and quantitative TLC methods have been described (30,63). The following chapter describes practical application of various procedures in a drug residue monitoring program.

Literature Cited

1. Schmidhofer, T.; Egli, H. R. Chimia 1974, 28, 424-9.
2. Stadhouders, J.; Hassing, F.; Galesloot, T. E. Neth. Milk Dairy J., 1981, 5, 23-33.
3. Horng, C.-B.; Hsieh, J.-T.; Ko, H.-C.; Jan, R.-H.; Li, J. H. Proc. Nat. Sci. Counc. Repub. China 1979, 3, 382-7.
4. Lott, A. F.; Vaughn, D. R. Soc. Appl. Bacteriol Tech. Ser. 1983, 18, 331-8.
5. Van Schothorst, M.; Van Leusden, F. Tijdschr. Diergeneeskd. 1974, 99, 880-2.
6. Tao, S. H.; Poumeyrol, M. Recl. Med. Vet. 1985, 161, 457-63.
7. Smither, R.; Vaughn, D. R. J. Appl. Bacteriol 1978, 44, 421-7.
8. Siewert, E.; Saga, B. VetMed-Ber. 1979, (1), 22p.; Chem. Abstr. 1980, 92, 39940.
9. Smither, R.; Lott, A. F.; Dalziel, A. W.; Ostler, D. C. J. Hyg. (Camb.) 1980, 85, 359-69.
10. Engel, W. W. B.; Van Leusden, F. W.; Nouws, J. F. M., in "Antimicrob. Agric., Proc. Int. Symp. Antibiot Agric.; Benefits Malefits," M. Woodbine, Ed. 4th 1983 (pub. 1984), 491-9.
11. Wagman, G. H.; Weinstein, M. J. "Chromatography of Antibiotics." J. Chromatogr. Libr. Vol. 26, Elsevier, New York, 1984.
12. Petz, M. Z. Lebensm. Unters.-Forsch. 1984, 180, 267-79.
13. Horwitz, W. J. Assoc. Off. Anal. Chem. 1981, 64, 104-30.
14. Tishler, F.; Sutter, J. L.; Bathish, J. N.; Hagman, H. E. J. Agric. Food Chem. 1968, 16, 50-53.
15. Matusik, J. E.; Barnes, C. J.; Newkirk, D. E.; Fazio, T. J. Assoc. Off. Anal. Chem., 1982, 65, 828-34.
16. Lloyd, W. E.; Jenny, A. L.; Cox, D. F.; Rotlinghaus, G. E. Amer. J. Vet. Res. 1981, 42, 339-43.
17. Terada, H.; Asanoma, M.; Tsubouchi, H. Eisei Kagaksu 1983, 29, 226-31; Chem. Abstr. 1984, 100, 50117.
18. Alawi, M. A.; Russel, H. A. Chromatographia 1981, 14, 704-6.
19. Patthy, M. J. Chromatogr. 1983, 275, 115-25.

20. Nakazawa, H.; Takabatake, E.; Hino, S.; Mtema, C. A. <u>Banseki Kagaku</u> 1983, 32, 179-83; Chem. Abstr. 1983, 98, 177573.
21. Parks, O. W. <u>J. Assoc. Off. Anal. Chem.</u> 1984, 67, 566-9.
22. Sakano, T.; Masuda, S.; Amano, T. <u>Chem. Pharm. Bull.</u> 1981, 29, 2290-5.
23. Seymour, D.; Rupe, B.D. <u>J. Pharm. Sci.</u> 1980, 69, 701-3.
24. Vilim, A. B.; Larocque, L.; MacIntosh, A. I. <u>J. Liq. Chromatogr.</u> 1980, 3, 1725-36.
25. Kishihara, S.; Skimokawa, C.; Izumi, H. <u>Ishikawa-ken Eisei Kogai Kenkyushu Nenpo</u> 1983, 20, 198-204; Chem. Abstr. 1984, 101, 165195.
26. Petz, M. <u>Z. Lebensm.-Unters. Forsch.</u> 1983, 176, 289-93.
27. Haagsma, N.; Nooteboom, R.J.; Gortemaker, B.G.M.; Maas, M.J. <u>Z. Lebensm.-Unters. Forsch.</u> 1985, 181, 194-7.
28. Haagsma, N.; Van de Water, C. <u>J. Chromatogr.</u> 1985, 333, 256-61.
29. Parks, O. W. <u>J. Assoc. Off. Anal. Chem.</u> 1982, 65, 632-4.
30. Thomas, M. H.; Soroka, K. E.; Thomas, S. H. <u>J. Assoc. Off. Anal. Chem.</u> 1983, 66, 881-3.
31. Thomas, M. H.; Epstein, R. L.; Ashworth, R. B.; Marks, H. <u>J. Assoc. Off. Anal. Chem.</u> 1983, 66, 884-92.
32. Haagsma, N.; Dieleman, B.; Gortemaker, B. G. M. <u>Tijdschr. Diergeneeskd.</u> 1984, 109, 8-12.
33. Schlatterer, B. <u>Z. Lebensm.-Unters. Forsch.</u> 1983, 176, 20-6.
34. Jonas, D.; Knapp, G.; Pollman, H. <u>Arch. Lebensmittelhyg.</u> 1983, 34, 138-41.
35. Haagsma, N. <u>Z. Lebensm.-Unters. Forsch.</u> 1985, 181, 45-6.
36. Stout, S. J.; Steller, W. A.; Manual, A. J.; Poeppel, M. O.; DaCunha, A. R. <u>J. Assoc. Off. Anal. Chem.</u> 1984, 67, 142-4.
37. Manuel, A. J.; Steller, W. A. <u>J. Assoc. Off. Anal. Chem.</u> 1981, 64, 794-9.
38. Garland, W; Miwa, B., Weiss, G.; Chen, G.; Saperstein, R.; MacDonald, A. <u>Anal. Chem.</u> 1980, 52, 842-6.
39. Paulson, G. D.; Mitchell, A. D.; Zaylskie, R. G. <u>J. Assoc. Off. Anal. Chem.</u> 1985, 68, 1000-6.
40. Suhre, F. B.; Simpson, R. M.; Shafer, J. W. <u>J. Agric. Food. Chem.</u> 1981, 29, 727-9.
41. Malanoski, A. J.; Barnes, C. J.; Fazio, T. <u>J. Assoc. Off. Anal. Chem.</u> 1981, 64, 1386-91.
42. Roach, J. A. G.; Sphon, J. A.; Hunt, D. F.; Crow, F. W. <u>J. Assoc. Off. Anal. Chem.</u> 1980, 63, 452-9.
43. Brumley, W. C.; Min, Z.; Matusik, J. E.; Roach, J. A. G.; Barnes, C. J.; Sphon, J. A.; Fazio, T. <u>Anal. Chem.</u> 1983, 55, 1405-9.
44. Giera, D. D.; Abdulla, R. F.; Occolowitz, J. L.; Dorman, D. E.; Mertz, J. L.; Sieck, R. F. <u>J. Agric. Food Chem.</u> 1982, 30, 260-3.
45. Schlatterer, B.; Weise, E. <u>Z. Lebensm.-Unters. Forsch.</u> 1982, 175, 392-8.
46. Allen, E. H. <u>J. Assoc. Off. Anal. Chem.</u> 1985, 68, 990-9.
47. Milhaut, G. <u>Ann. Rech. Vet.</u> 1985, 16, 133-48.
48. Bories, G. S. F.; Peleran, J.-C.; Wal, J.-M. <u>J. Assoc. Off. Anal. Chem.</u> 1983, 66, 1521-6.
49. Corry, J. E. L.; Sharma, M. R.; Bates, M. L. <u>Soc. Appl. Bact. Tech. Ser.</u> 1983, 18, 349-69.
50. Nouws, J. F. M. <u>Arch. Lebensmittelhyg.</u> 1981, 32, 103-10.

51. Bergner-Lang, B.; Kaechele, M. Deutsch. Lebensm.-Randsch. 1985, 81, 278-80.
52. Johannes, B.; Korfer, K. H.; Schad, J.; Ulbrich, I. Arch Lebensmittelhyg. 1983, 34, 1-7.
53. Moats, W. A. J. Chromatogr. (In press)
54. Ashworth, R. B. J. Assoc. Off. Anal. Chem. 1985, 68, 1013-8.
55. Ryan, J. J.; Dupont, J. A. J. Assoc. Off. Anal. Chem. 1974, 57, 828-31.
56. Sharma, J. P.; Bevill, R. F. J. Chromatogr. 1978, 166, 213-20.
57. Onji, Y.; Uno, M.; Fonigawa, K. J. Assoc. Off. Anal. Chem. 1984, 67, 1135-7.
58. Hamman, J.; Heeschen, W.; Toll, A. Milchwissensch. 1979, 34, 357-9.
59. Terada, H.; Asanoma, M.; Sakabe, Y. Eisei Kagaku 1984, 30, 138-48; Chem. Abstr. 1984, 101, 209188.
60. Hoshino, Y.; Horie, M.; Nose, N.; Iwasaki, H. Shokuhin Eiseigaku Zasshi 1984, 25, 430-5; Chem. Abstr. 1985, 102, 60866.
61. Oka, H.; Matsumoto, H.; Uno, K.; Harada, K; Kadowaki, S.; Suzuki, M.; J. Chromatogr. 1985, 325, 265-274.
62. Traldi, P.; Daolio, S.; Pelli, B.; Maffei Facino, R.; Carini, M. Biomed. Mass Spectrom. 1985, 12, 493-6.
63. Oka, H.; Uno, K.; Harada, K.; Suzuki, M. Yakugaku Zasshi 1983, 103, 531-7; Chem. Abstr. 1983, 99, 68865.
64. Botraglou, N.A.; Vassilopoulos, V. N.; Kufidis, D. E. Chem. Chron. 1984, 13, 37-44.
65. Juergens, U. Z. Lebensm.-Unters. Forsch. 1981, 173, 356-8.
66. Takeba, K.; Kanzaki, M.; Murakami, F.; Matsumoto, M. Kenkyu Nenpo - Tokyo-toritsu Eisei Kenkyusho 1984, 35, 187-91; Chem. Abstr. 1985, 102, 219712.
67. Nelis, H. J. C. F.; DeLeenheer, A. P. Clin. Chim. Acta 1980, 103, 209-17.
68. Mack, G. D.; Ashworth, R. B. J. Chromatogr. Sci. 1978, 16, 93-101.
69. Howell, H. R.; Rhodig, L. L.; Siegler, A. D. J. Assoc. Off. Anal. Chem. 1984, 67, 572-5.
70. Code of Federal Regulations, 21:556. U.S. Government Printing Office, Washington, D.C.
71. Hamman, J.; Tolle, A.; Blüthgen, A.; Heeschen, W. Milchwissensch. 1975, 30, 1-7.
72. Herbst, D. J. Food Prot. 1982, 45, 450-1.
73. Yoshimura, H.; Itoh, O.; Yonezawa, S. Jpn. J. Vet. Sci. 1981, 43, 833-40.
74. Rybinska, K. Rocz. Panstw. Zakl. Hig. 1980, 31, 177-80; Chem. Abstr. 1980, 93, 166197.
75. Moats, W. A. J. Agric. Food Chem. 1983, 31, 1348-50.
76. Bossuyt, R.; Van Rentergehm, R.; Waes, G. J. Chromatogr. 1976, 124, 37-42.
77. Munns, R. K.; Shimoda, W.; Roybal, J. E.; Vieira, C. J. Assoc. Off. Anal. Chem. 1985, 68, 968-71.
78. Moats, W. A. J. Agric. Food Chem. 1983, 31, 880-3.
79. Terada, H.; Sakabe, Y. J. Chromatogr. 1985, 348, 379-87.
80. Moats, W. A. J. Chromatogr. 1984, 317, 311-18.
81. Terada, H.; Asanoma, M.; Sakabe, Y. J. Chromatogr. 1985, 318, 299-306.

82. Moats, W. A.; Harris, E. W., Steele, N. C. **J. Agric. Food Chem.** (In press).
83. Uno, T.; Masada, M.; Kiyoshi, Y.; Terumichi, N. **Chem. Pharm. Bull.** 1981, 29, 1957-68.
84. Murai, Y.; Nakagawa, T.; Yamaoka, K.; Uno, T. **Chem. Pharm. Bull.** 1981, 29, 3290-7.
85. Moats, W. A. **J. Assoc. Off. Anal. Chem.** 1985, 68, 980-4.
86. Moats, W. A.; Harris, E. W.; Steele, N. C. **J. Assoc. Off. Anal. Chem.** 1985, 68, 413-16.
87. Weiss, G.; MacDonald, A. **J. Assoc. Off. Anal. Chem.** 1985, 68, 971-80.
88. Weiss, G.; Felicito, N. R.; Kaykaty, M.; Chen, G.; Caruso, A. Hargroves, E.; Crowley, C.; MacDonald, A. **J. Agric. Food Chem.** 1983, 31, 75-8.
89. Weiss, G.; Kaykaty, M.; Miwa, B. **J. Agric. Food Chem.** 1983, 31, 78-81.
90. Tikhova, D.; Peneva, V. **Vet.-Med. Nauki** 1982, 19, 52-6.; Chem. Abstr. 1982, 97, 180286.
91. Wojton, B.; Baran, E.; Dzialoszynska, J.; Michalski, M. **Med. Weter.** 1984, 40, 240-2.
92. Karkocha, I. **Rocz. Panstw. Zakl. Hig.** 1983, 39, 281-3.; Chem. Abstr. 1984, 100, 50105.
93. Shaikh, B.; Allen, E. H.; Gridley, J. C. **J. Assoc. Off. Anal. Chem.** 1985, 68, 29-36.
94. Lachatre, G.; Nicot, G.; Gannet, C.; Tronchet, J.; Merle, L.; Valette, J. P.; Nouaille, Y. **Analusis** 1983, 11, 168-77.
95. Kabra, P.M.; Bhatnagar, P. K.; Nelson, M. A. **J. Anal. Toxicol.** 1983, 7, 283-5.
96. Anon. **Food Chem. News** 1985, 27 (22), 21-2.
97. Munro, A. C.; Chaincy, M. G.; Wosoniecki, S. R. **J. Pharm. Sci.** 1978, 9, 1197-1204.
98. Kunin, C. M. **J. Infect. Dis.** 1970, 121, 55-64.
99. Wijkstroem, A.; Westerlund, D. **J. Pharm. Biomed. Anal.** 1983, 1, 293-9.
100. Cravedi, J. P.; Heuillet, G.; Peleran, J.-C.; Wal. J.-M. **Xenobiotica** 1985, 15, 115-21.
101. Wal, J. M.; Bories, C. F. **J. Antibiot.** 1973, 26, 687-91.
102. Hagestam, I. H.; Pinkerton, T. C. **Anal. Chem.** 1985, 57, 1757-63.

RECEIVED April 1, 1986

15

Pharmacokinetics and Residues of Sulfadimidine and Its N^4-Acetyl and Hydroxy Metabolites in Food-Producing Animals

J. F. M. Nouws[1], T. B. Vree[2], R. Aerts[3], and J. Grondel[4]

[1] R.V.V.-District 6, P. O. Box 40010, Nijmegen, the Netherlands
[2] Department of Clinical Pharmacy, Sint Radboud Hospital, Nijmegen, the Netherlands
[3] RIKILT, Wageningen, the Netherlands
[4] ZODIAC, University of Wageningen, the Netherlands

> Employing specific HPLC methods, the pharmacokinetics of sulfadimidine (SDM) and its metabolites N_4-acetyl (N_4-SDM), 6-hydroxymethyl (SCH_2OH), 5-hydroxy (SOH), and glucuronide (SOH-gluc.) were studied in various species. In general the SDM elimination half-lives depended on the metabolic rate and extent of metabolism as well as the renal excretion rate of the metabolites. N_4-SDM, SCH_2OH and SOH metabolites exhibited higher renal clearance values than SDM. Hydroxylation of SDM dominates in horses, calves, cows, and laying hens. The main metabolite in horses was SOH; in ruminants, SCH_2OH.
>
> In calves and cows at high dose levels (100 SDM mg/kg), a biphasic elimination SDM plasma concentration-time curve was observed with a steady state plasma SCH_2OH concentration resulting from the capacity limited hydroxylation of SDM into the latter. The drug concentrations in the milk reflected those in plasma. In calves and pigs, the SDM concentration in plasma exceeded that in muscle, kidney or liver tissue. The N_4-SDM tissue concentration was lower than that of SDM; in the calves' kidney, the SCH_2OH concentration exceeded that of SDM. In pigs, the acetylation pathway was predominant; no hydroxy metabolites could be detected in plasma and edible tissues. Eggs layed within 7 days after SDM therapy (100 mg SDM/kg/day) has been terminated show detectable quantities of the parent drug and its metabolites.

There are three main variables governing the pharmacokinetics of sulfonamides in animals, namely : 1) the molecular structure of the sulfonamide, 2) the mechanism and route of metabolism and 3) the renal excretion. By selecting one sulfonamide, e.g. sulfadimidine (SDM), for a comparative study, one is able to study species differences in metabolism, tissue disposition and renal clearances. Numerous reports discussing species differences in elimination half-lives for SDM as well as other sulfonamides, have been reviewed sulfadimidine in e.g. horses, pigs, ruminants, fowls, fish are obtained by the Bratton & Marshall method, which cannot distinguish SDM from its hydroxy metabolites.

Recently the hydroxy metabolites of various sulfonamides could be isolated and purified, so that specific HPLC techniques could be developed (22,23). As shown in Figure 1, sulfadimidine can be metabolized by hydroxylation at the 5 and 6 position of the pyrimidine ring and by the acetylation- deacetylation pathway (21). After hydroxylation, the metabolites may become glucuronidated and also acetylated (Figure 2). The hydroxy metabolites are microbiologically active and they can be potentiated by trimethoprim (13).

Because of its widespread therapeutic use and because the question of residues in food producing animals, SDM was selected for a study between species to compare its metabolism, the pharmacokinetics of the parent drug as well as its metabolites. Residue depletion studies were performed in edible tissues of calves, pigs and in the eggs of laying-hens.

MATERIAL AND METHODS

Drugs

Sodium sulfadimidine (33.3%) was obtained from A.U.V. (Cuyk,The Netherlands). N_4-acetylsulfadimidine (N_4-SDM), 6 -hydroxymethyl-sulfadimidine (SCH_2OH) and 5-hydroxysulfadimidine (SOH) were synthesized and isolated according Vree et al. (22,23).

Experiments

Animals were obtained from Mr. van Raay in Gassel, the Central Animal Laboratory at the University of Nijmegen, Large Animal Clinics at the University of Utrecht, and from Zodiac at the Agricultural University of Wageningen, the Netherlands.

SDM was administered either intravenously, intramuscularly, orally, or intraperitoneally to horses, calves, cows, pigs, laying-hens and carp. Heparinized blood samples were taken at regular time intervals, centrifuged and plasma was deep frozen at -20 C pending HPLC analysis. Urine was collected by either spontaneous voiding, catheterisation, or with special collection urine and feces facilities for the horses, ruminants, and pigs. When the pigs and calves were slaughtered, specimens of kidney, liver, muscle, plasma, and urine were sampled and prepared as described (16). The eggs of laying hens were collected during SDM administration and for the 14 days post administration. For the carp, water samples were taken at 4 to 12 h intervals, after which the water was changed.

HPLC Analysis

Deglucuronidation, sample preparation and HPLC analysis were performed as described elsewhere (14,15,16).

SDM, its N_4-SDM, and two hydroxymetabolites were determined simultaneously in the several test specimen.

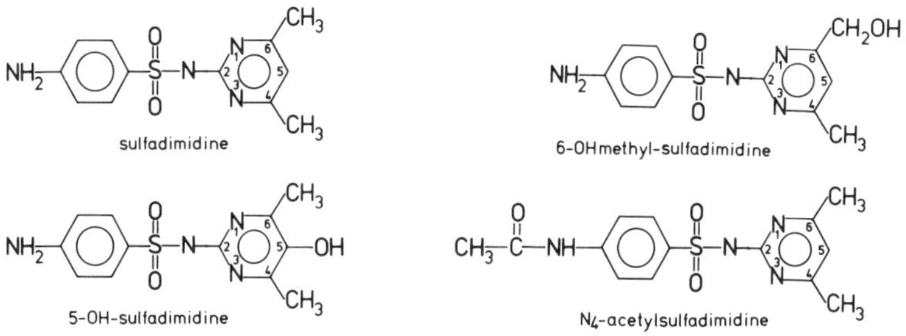

Figure 1. Molecular structures of sulfadimidine (SDM), its 5-hydroxy-4,6-dimethyl-pyrimidine (SOH), its 6-hydroxymethyl-4-methyl-pyrimidine (SCH_2OH) and its N_4-acetyl metabolite (N_4-SDM).

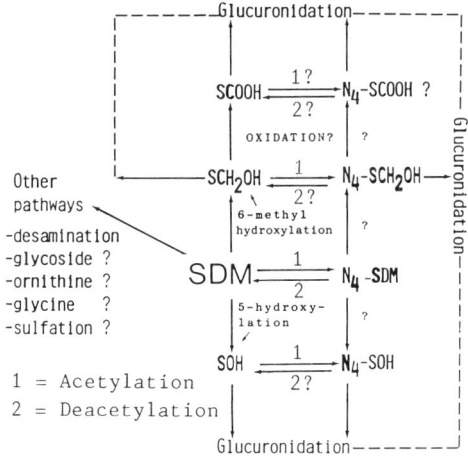

Figure 2. Metabolic pathways of sulfadimidine.

RESULTS

Table I summarizes the percentages of sulfadimidine and its metabolites in the plasma of the different species; Table II shows the tissue to plasma drug concentration ratios for SDM and its metabolites, while Table III presents the urinary recovery data (for poultry urinary plus faecal recovery). The metabolic pathways observed in various species are summarized in a scheme (Figure 2). Selected data obtained are illustrated in Figures 3 - 9.

Horses

In the horse, hydroxylation is more important than acetylation as a metabolic pathway, with hydroxylation at the 5 position being dominant over hydroxylation of the 6-methyl group. Low percentages of metabolites are present in plasma, for N_4-SDM, 0.6 to 0.9 %; for SCH_2OH, 0.38 to 0.71 %; and for SOH, 0.38 to 6.7 %. The plasma concentration-time curves of the metabolites run parallel to that of SDM. The elimination half-life of sulfadimidine varies between 5 and 14 h. The main metabolite in urine, accounting for 50 % of the drugs present (Table III), is the SOH and its glucuronide.

Cows and calves

SDM is extensively hydroxylated into hydroxy derivatives and to a lesser extent acetylated into N_4-SDM. Hydroxylation of the 6-methyl group to form 6-hydroxymethylsulfadimidine dominates (1.5 times) hydroxylation at the 5 position (Table III). At high dosage levels (100 -200 mg/kg), a biphasic elimination SDM plasma concentration-time curve was observed with a steady state plasma concentration of SCH_2OH (6-15 µg/ml) during the period in which the SDM plasma concentration exceeded 20 µg/ml. A capacity limited hydroxylation of SDM into SCH_2OH was noticed in ruminant calves and cows at a dosage level of 100-200 mg/kg (15). An unknown metabolite (X) and its glucuronide was detected either in the plasma (Figure 3) or urine of cows, goats, and horses (Table I and III). The unknown metabolite (X) may be the further oxidation product of the 6-hydroxymethyl metabolite. In which case it was tentatively assumed to be 6-carboxysulfadimidine and its glucuronide. (In calculating the concentration of the unknown metabolite, which eluted from the HPLC column just before the 5-hydroxy metabolite (SOH), the molar extinction of SOH was used). This unknown metabolite did not penetrate the udder (Figure 4) presumably because of its polar nature. The N_4-SDM plasma concentrations run parallel to SDM beyond 4 h after injection at all dosages in all animals.

In milk, the concentration of SDM and its metabolites was a reflection of those in plasma (14; Figure 4). The disposition of SDM in plasma, edible tissues, bile and urine of calves are illustrated in Figure 5. As shown, the SDM concentration in plasma was higher than that in the edible tissues. The latter is also confirmed by the tissue to plasma concentration ratios of SDM and its metabolites which were lower than 1, except for the metabolite ratios in kidney tissue (Table II). The SCH_2OH concentration in the kidney exceeded those of SDM (Figure 6). The N_4-SDM metabolite concentrations in muscle, kidney and liver were always below those of SDM (Table II;

Table I MEAN PERCENTAGES[1] OF SULFADIMIDINE AND ITS METABOLITES IN PLASMA OF DIFFERENT SPECIES.

SPECIES	Dose mg/kg	% SDM	% N_4-SDM	% SCH_2OH	% SOH	% $X_{(+gluc.)}$	Reference
Man (S)[a]	12	57.6	32.7	—	—	—	
(F)	12	23.5	67.3	—	—	—	
Calf	10	62.6	5.7	30.9	1.4	—	15
	100	79.7	11.0	8.6	0.7	—	15
Cow	10	70.5	2.1	22.4	3.9	3.4	15
	100	85.4	2.3	9.7	1.0	2.2	15
Goat	100	77.6	1.5	7.2	5.4	8.5	17
Horse	20–200	95.0	0.7	0.5	3.8	—	
Pigs	20	90.0	10.0	—	—	—	16
Poultry	100	87.8	7.5	4.5	1.2	—	
Fish(carp)	560	96.8	2.8	0.4	0.05	—	

(a) S = slow acetylator phenotype; F = fast acetylator phenotype.
1) Percentage of AUC vs total AUC (= AUC parent + metabolites).

Table II CONCENTRATION RATIO'S OF SULFADIMIDINE AND ITS METABOLITES BETWEEN TISSUE SPECIMEN AND PLASMA.

Drug concentration in specimen vs. plasma	SDM	SCH_2OH	SOH	N_4-SDM
Calves	Mean and standard deviation[a].			
Kidney vs plasma	0.34+0.18 (n=11)	1.89+1.18 (n=12)	4.76+1.14 (n=4)	2.50+0.54 (n=3)
Muscle) vs plasma homogenate)	0.38+0.18 (n=10)	0.36+0.10 (n=4)	0.18+0.02 (n=3)	0.20+0.04 (n=4)
Muscle drip vs plasma	0.39+0.20 (n=10)	0.32+0.02 (n=5)	0.23+0.13 (n=4)	0.38+0.06 (n=4)
Liver vs plasma	0.24+0.18 (n=7)	0.27+0.13 (n=3)	0.31+0.20 (n=3)	0.43+0.18 (n=3)
Pigs				
Kidney vs plasma	0.29+0.06 (n=10)	—	—	1.26+0.67 (n=9)
Muscle homogenate vs plasma	0.19+0.08 (n=10)	—	—	0.38+0.23 (n=10)
Muscle drip vs plasma	0.42+0.15 (n=11)	—	—	0.45+0.23 (n=10)
Liver vs plasma	0.15+0.12 (n=8)	—	—	0.33+0.30 (n=4)

a = Number of samples in parentheses.
— = absent

Table III PLASM ELIMINATION HALF-LIFE, AND URINARY RECOVERY OF SULFADIMIDINE AND ITS METABOLITES EXPRESSED AS PERCENTAGES OF THE DOSE ADMINISTERED (mean values) IN DIFFERENT SPECIES.

SPECIES	Dose mg/kg	$T_{1/2el}$ hours	Time period in hours	URINARY RECOVERY			EXPRESSED AS PERCENTAGE OF THE DOSE			
				Total recovery	%SDM	$%N_4$-SDM	$%SCH_2OH$	%SOH (+gluc)	%X	$%X_{gluc}$
Calf	10	3.5	0-72	84	7	13	50	14	—	—
	100	15+5[a]	0-120	88	22	34	26	6	—	—
Cow	10	3.5	0-72	86	9.7	7.2	50.5	18.0	—	4.8
	100	12+6.5[a]	0-72	72	26	9	26	8	0.2	2.3
Pigs	20	9-14	0-140	77.8	13.4	41.0	18.7[b]	4.7	—	—
Goat	100	2.7-3.8	0-20	98	15.1	4.5	28.2	30.9	1.4	18.2
Horse	200	9.5	0-27	25	10.1 (40.5[c])	1.4 (5.6)	0.25 (1.0)	12.7 (51)	0.4 (1.4)	—
Fish (carp)	560	17.5	0-48	64.4	62.2	1.8	0.23	0.18	—	—
Man (S)[d]	12	7.7	0-60	88	12.9	62.5	6.3	3.5	2.8	—
(F)	12	1.6+5[a]	0-60	87	3.6	74.1	7.0	0.75	1.56	—
Poultry	100	10+3.5[a]	0-60	42	13.9	12.1	10.2	5.8	—	—

— = not detected
a) biphasic elimination-time curve (both elimination half-lives given).
b) present as an acetylated derivative.
c) relative percentage of the total recovered drug in 27 h in parenthesis
d) S = slow acetylator phenotype;   F = fast acetylator phenotype

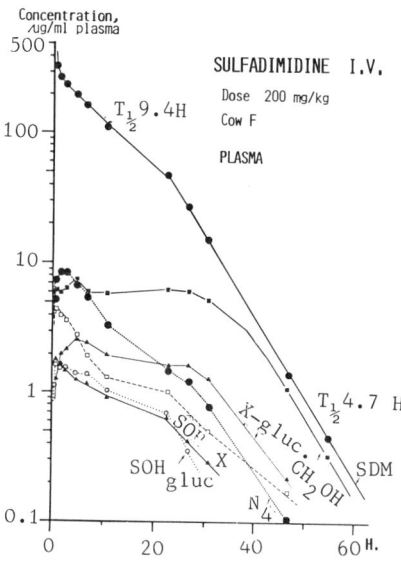

Figure 3. Plasma concentration-time curves of sulfadimidine (SDM), and its 6-methylhydroxy (CH_2OH), 5-hydroxy (SOH) and its glucuronide (SOH_{gluc}), N_4-acetyl (N_4) and unknown (X) metabolites in a cow after an intravenous dose of 200 mg/kg sulfadimidine.

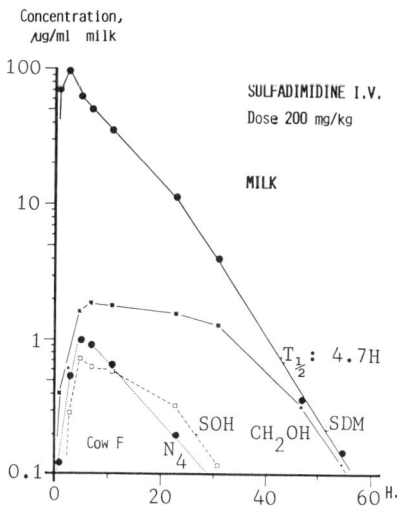

Figure 4. Disposition of sulfadimidine (SDM), its 6-methylhydroxy (CH_2OH), 5-hydroxy (SOH) and N_4-acetyl (N_4) metabolites in milk of a dairy cow following intravenous administration of 200 mg SDM/kg.

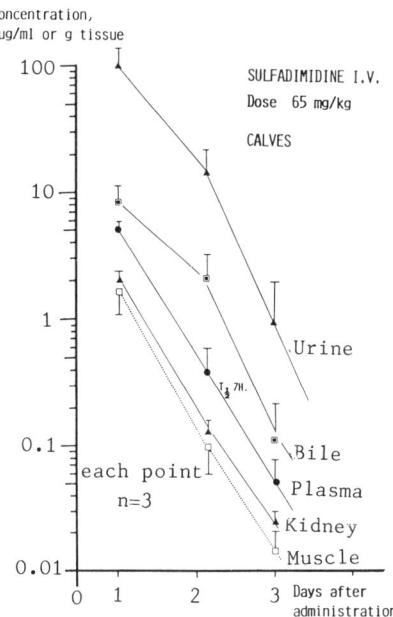

Figure 5. Disposition of sulfadimidine in urine, bile, plasma and tissues of calves following intravenous administration of 65 mg/kg intravenously.

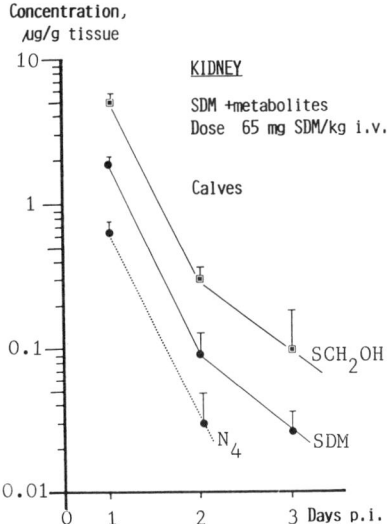

Figure 6. Disposition of sulfadimidine(SDM), 6-methylhydroxy (CH$_2$OH), and N$_4$-acetylsulfadimidine (N$_4$) in the kidney of calves following intravenous administration of 65 mg SDM/kg.

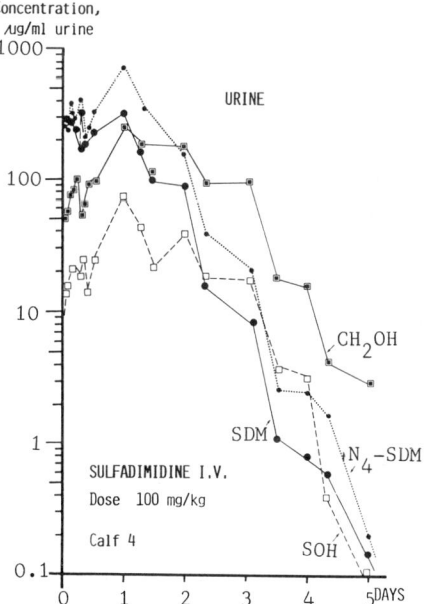

Figure 7. Urine concentration-time curves of sulfadimidine (SDM), and its metabolites (N$_4$, CH$_2$OH, SOH) in urine of a calf following intravenous administration of 100 mg SDM/kg.

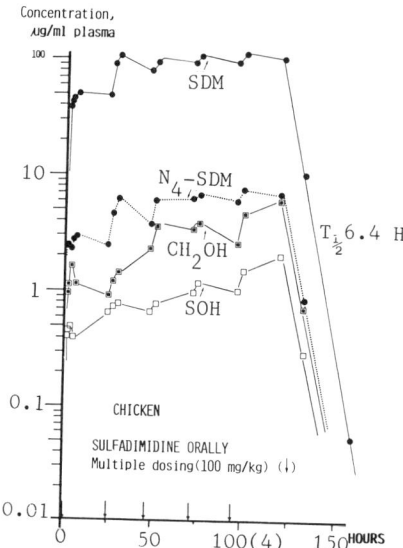

Figure 8. Plasma disposition of sulfadimidine (SDM), its 6-methylhydroxy (CH_2OH), 5-hydroxy (SOH) and N_4-acetyl (N_4) metabolites in plasma of a laying-hen during and after cessation of multiple oral dosing of 100 mg SDM/kg/day during 5 days.

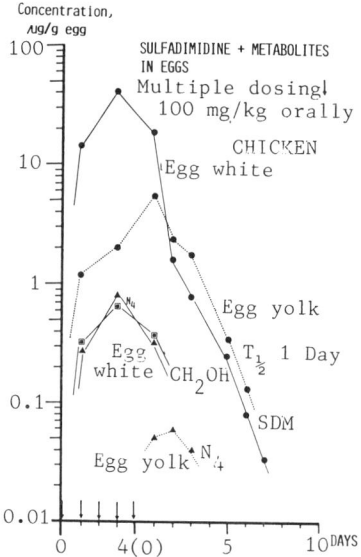

Figure 9. Drug depletion time curves of sulfadimidine (SDM), and its metabolites (N_4, CH_2OH) in the egg albumen and egg yolk during and after cessation of the administration of 100 mg SDM/kg during 5 days.

In calves and cows, SDM was excreted by glomerular filtration minus tubular reabsorption; its renal clearance was urine flow correlated, and amounts to half of the creatinine clearance. The SCH_2OH hydroxy metabolite was excreted by glomerular filtration and partly by tubular secretion, whereas both N_4-SDM and SOH were excreted predominantly by tubular secretion (15). The main metabolite in urine SCH_2OH was 23 to 55 % of the administered dose (Table III). The urine concentration-time curves for SDM and its metabolites are illustrated in Figure 7 for a high SDM dosage.

Pigs
In pigs SDM is metabolised by acetylation into N_4-SDM. The SCH_2OH hydroxy metabolite was excreted as an acetylated derivative; SCH_2OH itself could not be detected in plasma, edible tissues and urine. At a dosage level of 20 mg/kg, traces of SOH could be only detected in the urine (Table III; ref.16). The N_4-SDM plasma concentration-time curve was parallel to the SDM curve. The elimination half-life ranged from 9 to 14 hours (5,16). In pigs the N_4-SDM percentage (vs total drug concentration) in plasma and edible tissues was relatively higher than in calves, but the N_4-SDM distribution pattern was similar in these two species (Table II). The highest N_4-SDM concentrations were found in plasma, kidney, muscle and liver, respectively. The renal clearance of N_4-SDM was three times higher than that of creatinine, that of the parent drug is 7 times less than the creatinine clearance (16). Depending on the dosage level, SDM residues in edible tissues could be detected 7 to 14 days post administration (5,16).

Poultry
Laying-hens eliminate sulfadimidine rapidly by metabolic pathways including hydroxylation and acetylation. Following intravenous SDM administration, a biphasic elimination-time curve was noticed ($T_{1/2}$: 10.2 + 3.3 H). Figure 8 shows the plasma disposition of SDM and its metabolites following an oral SDM bolus administration once daily of 100 mg/kg to a chicken. The percentage of N_4-SDM in plasma is the highest (Table I). Within 3 days of termination of the SDM therapy, plasma concentrations of SDM and its metabolites falls rapidly below the detection limit of the HPLC method (0.02 μg/ml).

In eggs an increase of SDM in the albumen as well as in the yolk occurrred during the drug administration period. SDM residues could be detected in the eggs layed 7 days post the cessation of the administration. Traces of the N_4-SDM and hydroxy metabolites were detectable till 3 days post SDM administration (Figure 9).

Approximately 16 % of the dose is hydroxylated, 5.8 % at the 5 position (SOH) and 10.2 % at 6 position (SCH_2OH). No glucuronide metabolites were formed. Acetylation accounted for 12.7 % of the dose, while the recovery of the parent drug was 13.9 %. Thus approximately 58 % of the administered dose is lost after i.v. application (Table III). The renal clearance of the hydroxy and acetylated metabolites were 10 to 50 fold higher than that of SDM.

Fish (Carp)
In the carp, SDM is hydroxylated and acetylated only to a small extent (Table III). The main metabolite is N_4-SDM; only 2 % of the

0.18 % is excreted as SOH and 0.23 % as SCH_2OH (Table III). The clearance values of SDM, N_4-SDM and the hydroxy metabolites were equivalent and the elimination was predominantly by a passive diffusion process (9).

DISCUSSION

In mammals, all N_4-acetyl metabolites formed at low and high dosages as well as hydroxy metabolites formed at low dosages show plasma concentration-time curves that are parallel to that of the parent SDM. This observation means that the intrinsic elimination of the metabolites is higher than that of the parent drug (23). The hydroxy metabolites are eliminated partly by glomerular filtration minus tubular reabsorption, and partly by tubular secretion, the net result being equal to 10 times higher than the renal clearance of the parent sulfadimidine. The N_4-acetyl and glucuronides are eliminated predominantly by tubular secretion. In fish (carp), the plasma clearance of SDM and its metabolites occur to the same extent, presumably by a passive diffusion process (glomerular filtration or diffusion across the gills (9).

In mammals and fowls, the metabolism of sulfadimidine means that the parent drug is converted into a form that can be excreted faster than the parent. Thus hydroxylation, the subsequent conjugation and as acetylation speed up the elimination of SDM. In dwarf goats (17), cows, calves, and chickens, hydroxylation of the 6-methyl group (SCH_2OH) dominates that at the 5 position (SOH). In goats the hydroxylation rate is greater than in calves and cows (17); in the latter a capacity limited hydroxylation of SDM into SCH_2OH was observed at a dosage of 100- 200 mg SDM/kg. A similar capacity limited elimination of SDM was reported for SDM at a dosage of 200 mg/kg in goats (mixed breeds) by Van Gogh (8), for sulfadiazine in rabbits (20) and for sulfamonomethoxine in pigs (19). Between goat breeds (and presumably also in other species) hydroxylator phenotypes exist. In horses the hydroxylation at the 5 position (SOH) dominates over that of the 6-methyl group (SCH_2OH). A longer elimination half-life was noticed in this species. Thus the rate and yield of hydroxylation as well as the renal clearance values determine the elimination half-life in those species for which hydroxylation dominates the acetylation pathway (e.g. in cows, calves, goats, and horses).

In chickens a pattern similar to a capacity limited-elimination was noticed. The cause may be either a capacity limitation in the SDM metabolism (hydroxylation?) of SDM or extensive drug reabsorption from the cloaca occurring at night(known as chrono-pharmacokinetics). In the chicken, 58 % of the intravenously administered dose is lost, which is also reported for other birds (24). Thus birds must possess additional metabolic pathways.

When hydroxylation is absent or negligible, both the position of the acetylation-deacetylation equilibrium and the renal excretion rate determine the elimination half-life. This can be exemplified by comparing the SDM disposition in pigs and man. The renal clearance values of N_4-SDM in both species are the same (approximately 10 ml/min/kg), but in man the equilibrium favours the acetylated

Therefore the yield of N_4-SDM formed and excreted per min. (excretion rate) is higher in man than in pigs resulting in man in shorter elimination half-lives ($T_{1/2}$:2 to 7 h vs. 9 to 14 h for pigs). The acetylation-deacetylation equilibrium is not affected by dosage: the same plasma concentration ratios between N_4-SDM and SDM were measured in cows at 10 and 200 mg/kg dose level. However the renal clearance of N_4-SDM is diminished at the high dosage of 100-200 mg/kg. At high SDM dosage, acetylation becomes relatively more important in the elimination process of SDM (Table III). Finally, differences in elimination half-lives between species cannot be correlated to differences in plasma protein binding data.

SDM and its metabolites are poorly distributed and no accumulation in edible tissues is observed. The metabolite concentrations are lower than those of SDM, except for SCH_2OH in the kidney of calves. The SDM concentrations in urine exceed those of plasma. Thus employing the urine or the pre-urine present in the renal pelvis as a test specimen, sulfonamide sensitive bioassays would be highly suitable for monitoring slaughtered animals (13). The advantages of the bioassay methods are the sensitivity for a wide spectrum of antibacterial drugs, the ease of performing the analysis and the low cost. Furthermore the shortcomings in the bioassays can be counterbalanced by selected physical chemical methods, e.g. RIA, ELISA-techniques, HPLC, etc.(3).

With respect to SDM administration to egg laying poultry, a withholding time of 7 days has to be considered. During the drug administration an increase of the SDM concentration in eggs (yolk and albumen) is noticed. This feature has been already reported by Blom (6) and for other drugs (3,25), which can be explained by drug absorbtion during the explosive growth of the egg follicle (egg-yolk) in the third development stage (1,7). The permeability of the follicle seems to change during the various stages in development of the ovum and in the final stage (last nine days before ovulation) phosfolipides are mainly deposited in the yolk. The highest drug concentration in the egg yolk are found 4 to 6 days after the onset of drug administration (1). The albumen (egg white) is formed in a relative short period (20-24 h before laying). The occurrence and level of the drug in the albumen is primarily related to the physical chemical properties of the drug and plasma drug concentrations in the last 24 h period before laying (1).

In conclusion, differences in the persistence and pharmacokinetics of SDM (and presumably for sulfonamides in general) between species depend on:
1. the extent and rate of hydroxylation, conjugation , acetylation as well as deacetylation, which differ between species and which is presumably related to the sulfonamide structure.
2. the renal clearance values of the metabolites, which may be quite constant between species and which depend on the chemical structure.
3. the position of the acetylation-deacetylation equilibrium.
4. in ruminants: the dosage.
5. other factors affecting absorption and elimination of SDM such as age of the animal(15), breed, disease state of the animal (2,17), composition of the food, time of year(10), mode of application, and formulation aspects(4).

Literature Cited

1. Anhalt,G. Arch. Geflügelk.1977,41,232-237.
2. Anika,S.M., Nouws,J.F.M.,Van Duin,C.T.M.,Van Miert,A.S. J.P.A.M. In"Comparative Veterinary Pharmacology and Therapy, 3rd EAVPT congress,Ghent". Part I: Abstracts,1985,p.216.
3. Arnold,D.,Berg,D.von, Boertz,A.K., Mallick,U., Somogyi,A. Arch. Lebensmittelhyg.1984,35, 131-136.
4. Bevill,R.F., Dittert,L.W., Bourne,D.W.A. J. pharmac. Sci. 1977,66,619-622.
5. Biehl,L.G., Bevill,R.F., Limpoka,M., Koritz,G.D. J. vet. Pharmacol. Therap. 1981,4, 285-290.
6. Blom,L. Acta vet. Scand. 1975, 16, 396-404.
7. Gilbert,A.B. In " Physiology and biochemistry of the domestic fowl.", Bell,D.J., and Freeman,B.M. Eds. Academic Press, New York,1971;Vol.III,Chap. 50,54,56.
8. Gogh,H.van J. vet. Pharmacol. Ther. 1980,3,69-81.
9. Haenen,O.L.M., Grondel,J.L. and Nouws,J.F.M. (1985) In"Comparative Veterinary Pharmacology ,Toxicology and Therapy, 3 rd EAVPT congress,Ghent", 1985,Part I: Abstracts, p.112.
10. Nawaz,M. Vet. Rec.1983, 112, 379-381.
11. Nielsen,P. Biochem. J.1973,136,1039-1045.
12. Nouws,J.F.M., Vree,T.B., Hekster, Y. The Veterinary Quarterly 1985,7,70-72.
13. Nouws,J.F.M., Driessens,F., Smulders,A., Vree,T.B. The veterinary Quarterly 1985, 7, 76-78.
14. Nouws,J.F.M., Vree,T.B., Breukink,H.J., Baakman,M., Driessens,F., Smulders,A. The veterinary Quarterly 1985, 7,177-186.
15. Nouws,J.F.M., Vree,T.B., Baakman,M., Driessens,F., H.J.Breukink, Mevius, D. Am. J. Vet. Res.,1986,in press.
16. Nouws,J.F.M., Vree,T.B., Baakman,M., Driessens,F., Vellenga,L., Mevius,D. The veterinary Quarterly,1986,8, in press.
17. Nouws,J.F.M., Anika,S.M., Miert,A.S.J.P.A.M., Vree,T.B., Baakman,M., Duin,C.T. Res. Vet. Sci.,1986, in press.
18. Oikawa,H., Nakamoto,K., Hirota,K., Katagiri,K. Poultry Sci., 1977,56, 813-21.
19. Shimode,M., Shimizu,T., Kokue,E., Hayama,T. Jpn. J. vet. Sci. 1984,46,331-337.
20. Souich,P. du, McLean,A.J., Lalka,D., Vicuna,N., Chauhuri,E., McNay,J.L. J. Pharmac. exp. Ther. 1978,207, 228-235.
21. Vree,T.B.,Tijhuis,M.,Baakman,M., Hekster,Y.A., Biomed. Mass Spectrom. 1983, 10,114-119.
22. Vree.T.B., Tijhuis,M., Nouws,J.F.M., Hekster,Y.A. Pharmac. Weekbl., Sci. Ed. 1984, 6,80-87.
23. Vree,T.B., Hekster,Y.A., Tijhuis,M. In"Pharmacokinetics of sulfonamides revisited." Eds. T.B.Vree and Y.A.Hekster. Antibiotics and Chemotherapy 1985,34,5-65.
24. Vree,T.B.,Hekster,Y.A., Nouws,J.F.M., Dorrestein,G.M. In "Pharmacokinetics of sulfonamides revisited". T.B.Vree & Y.A. Hekster Eds. Antibiotics and Chemotherapy 1985,34, 130-170.
25. Yoshida,M.D., Kubota,D., Yonezawa,S., Nakamura,H., Yamaoka,R., Yoshimura,H. Jap. Poult. Sci. 1973,10, 254-260.

RECEIVED February 18, 1986

INDEXES

Author Index

Aerts, R., 168
Argauer, Robert J., 35
Brown, Jeffrey, 137
Burg, R. W., 61
Frappaolo, Philip J., 100
Grondel, J., 168
Gustafson, Richard H., 1
Hays, Virgil W., 74
Jukes, Thomas H., 112
Katz, Stanley E., 142
Livingston, Robert C., 128
Misra, Arun K., 49
Moats, William A., 154
Nouws, J. F. M., 168
Schultze, W. D., 23
Schwab, Bernard, 137
Shahani, Khem M., 88
Vree, T. B., 168
Whalen, Paul J., 88
Ziv, G., 8

Subject Index

A

Absorption of antimicrobial agents, influencing factors, 15
Acidophilin, food preservative, 94,95t
Agglutination
  application, 150
  description, 149-150
American foulbrood control
  oxytetracycline, 36-45
  sulfathiazole, 36,37f
Amikacin, use in food animals, 19
Aminoglycoside detection, by chromatographic methods, 163
Aminoglycosides
  description, 18-19
  future development, 18
  use as feed additives, 4
Analysis of risks of antibiotics in animal feeds
  effects on animal health, 108-109
  impact of ban of subtherapeutic use, 109
  mortality rate estimates, 107-108
  petition on subtherapeutic uses, 106
Animal health products
  anthelmintic, 68-69
  anticoccidials, 66-67
  classification of agents, 62t
  feed additives, 62-65
  growth promotants, 65-66
  market, 62
Anthelmintic agents, 68-69
Antibacterial feed additives, synthetic and antibiotic, 3t
Antibacterial therapy, objective, 12
Antibiotic combinations, advantages and disadvantages, 21

Antibiotic feed additives, antibiotic resistance controversy, 5-6
Antibiotic growth effect
  characteristics, 113t
  vs. contamination, 113,114t
  vs. disease level, 114-115t
Antibiotic residues
  analysis by microbiological assay methods, 142-151
  tests, 139-141
Antibiotic residues in foods, identification by physicochemical methods, 154-163
Antibiotic use in meat production, extent of agricultural use, 5
Antibiotics
  anthelmintic agent, 68-69
  anticoccidials, 62
  definition, 2,49,74
  feed additives, 62-65
  growth promotion, 56
  higher plants as source, 54-56
  history in animal health, 62
  legislation, 56
  products for parenteral or topical administration to animals, 62,63t
  properties as feed additives, 2
  registration and commercialization, 1-3
  rumen additives 67-68
  selection, 11-13
  therapeutic uses, 8-21
  treatment of mastitis, 23-32
  usage in animals, 62t,74-75
  uses in animal agriculture, 3-5
  uses in drinking water formulations, 4-5
  uses as injectables, 4-5

INDEX

Antibiotics in agriculture, regulatory aspects, 128-136
Antibiotics in animal feeds
  animal welfare, 124
  approved drugs, 116
  approved levels, 116-117
  bacterial resistance, 118-124
  effect on children, 124
  effect of low levels, 112-125
  effect on resistance, 116
  risks to human health, 100-109
  theories against usage, 124-125
Antibiotics in animal production
  bacterial resistance, 77-78,80-85
  benefits, 92-96
  effect of antibiotic residues, 78
  effect of residual antibiotics, 91-92,93t
  effect of resistant microorganisms, 89,90t,91
  effect of subtherapeutic use on human health, 78-79
  impact of antibiotic restrictions, 79-80
  reasons for usage, 75-76t,77
  risk to humans, 88
  types, 75
  uses, 89
Antibiotics as crop protectants
  bacterial control, 51-52
  examples, 50,51t,54t
  fungal disease control, 50-52
  mycoplasmal disease control, 53,55t
  plant virus disease control, 52-54
Anticoccidials
  lasalocid, 66
  monensin, 66-67
Antimicrobial agents, types, 16-21
Antimicrobial therapy for mastitis
  aim, 31
  effectiveness against mastitis, 31
Antimicrobials, development as feed additives, 1-6
Apramycin, use in food animals, 19
Assays for antibiotic residues in milk
  colorimetric assay for β-lactams, 148t
  disc assay, 147
  penzyme test, 148
Aureomycin, growth-promoting effect, 113
Avermectins
  activity, 68-69
  discovery, 68

B

Bacterial control, by antibiotics, 51-52

Bacterial resistance to antibiotics
  effect on humans, 77-78,82-84
  effect on intestinal bacteria, 118
  effect of medical practice, 119-120
  effect of short-term therapeutic use, 81-82
  effect of time, 123-124
  influencing factors, 80,81t
  reduction of human exposure, 85
  report, 119-120
  Salmonella, 118-123
  types, 77
  virulence, 84-85
Beekeeping, use of antibiotics, 35-46
Benefits of antibiotics
  livestock production, 92-93
  naturally occurring antibiotics in foods, 93-96

C

Calf antibiotic-sulfonamide test, description, 140
Cephalosporins, use in food animals, 17-18
Chemotherapeutics, definition, 74
Chloramphenicol, description, 20
Chloramphenicol detection, by chromatographic methods, 158
Chromatographic methods for residue determination
  aminoglycoside detection, 163
  chloramphenicol detection, 158
  ionophore detection, 162
  β-lactam antibiotic detection, 159,160-161t,162
  macrolide antibiotic detection, 162
  sulfonamide detection, 155,156-157t,158
  tetracycline detection, 158-159
Clinical mastitis, definition, 26
Colorimetric assay for β-lactams
  description of delvotest, 148
  interpretation of delvotest results, 148t
  limits of detection, 148t
Competitive receptor assays
  applications, 146-147
  description of Charm test, 146
  limits of detection and measurement of antibiotics, 147t
Compound evaluation system, monitoring chemicals, 138
Consumption factor, values, 130t
Crop protection, antibiotic usage, 49-56
Cup-plate (well) procedure, 143
Cylinder-plate procedure, description, 143

D

Diethylstilbesterol, growth promotant, 65-66
Diffusion systems
  advantages and disadvantages, 143-144
  description, 143
  detection and measurement levels of residues, 144t
  influencing factors, 144
  interferences, 145
  maximum sensitivity, 144-145
  types, 143
Disc assay, description, 147
Dosage determination of antibiotics
  dosage schedule, 12-13
  minimal inhibitory drug concentrations, 12
  serum or tissue level, 12
  subinhibitory drug concentration, 13
  variables affecting dosage, 13
Dry cow therapy for mastitis
  advantages, 28
  antibiotic formulations, 28
  description, 24,26
  efficacy, 28,29t
  prophylactic efficacy, 30-31

E

Enzyme-linked immunosorbent assays
  antibody inhibition, 151
  direct competition, 151
  double-antibody sandwich, 151
Enzyme multiplied immunoassay technique, description, 151
Erythromycin, use as feed additives, 4
Exploratory sampling, description, 138

F

Feed additives
  antibacterial, 3t
  antibiotics, 62,64t
  benefits, 64
  categories, 2t
  discovery, 62-63
  foreign market, 65,66t
  growth permittants, 62-64,65t
  properties, 2
  registration and commercialization, 1-3
  risks to human health, 64
Fermentation products
  classification of agents used on plants, 69t

Fermentation products--Continued
  market for plant usage, 69,71
  usage on plants, 69,70t,71
Finite tolerance, definition, 129t
First-generation cephalosporins, description, 17
Fluoroimmunoassays, description, 150-151
Food and Drug Administration, responsibilities, 137
Fumagillin, control of Nosema apis, 45-46
Fungal disease control, by antibiotics, 50-52

G

Gentamicin, use in food animals, 19
Gram-positive antibiotics, use as feed additives, 4
Growth promotants, 65-66

H

Health risk of antibiotics in animal feeds
  analysis, 106-109
  historical perspective, 101-103
  recent studies, 103-104
  risk factors, 105-106
Herd medication
  advantages and disadvantages, 10
  prophylactic treatment, 10-11
High-voltage electrophoresis for residue determination, advantages and disadvantages, 154-155
Honeybee larvae, susceptibility to American foulbrood, 35

I

Immunological systems
  antibody production, 149
  basic reaction, 149
  description, 148-149
  techniques for antibody analysis, 149-151
Infectious resistance, definition, 120
Ionophore detection, by chromatographic methods, 162

INDEX

K

Kanamycin, use in food animals, 19

L

β-Lactam antibiotic detection, by chromatographic methods, 159,160-161t,162
Lactational therapy for mastitis
  effectiveness, 27
  products, 26-27
Lactic acid bacteria
  antibiotic production, 94,95t,96
  usage in food preservation, 93,94t
Legislation, antibiotic usage for plant protection, 56
Levels of antibiotics
  effect of cooking, 117-118
  sensitivity, 117-118
  withdrawal time, 117-118
Live animal swab test, description, 139

M

Macrolides, description, 19
Marker residue, definition, 134
Mastitis
  causes and treatment, 23-24
  cost, 23
  definition, 23
Mastitis control
  dry cow therapy, 28-31
  lactational therapy, 26-27
  selective dry cow therapy, 28,30
Mastitis pathogens
  dry cow therapy, 24,26
  sensitivity to antibiotics, 24,25t
Meat production, extent of antibiotic use, 5
Microbiological assay methods
  advantages and disadvantages, 142-143
  antibiotic residues in milk, 147
  colorimetric assay for β-lactams, 148t
  competitive receptor assays, 146-147
  diffusion systems, 143-145
  immunological systems, 148-151
  turbidimetric systems, 145-146
Microlide antibiotic detection, by chromatographic methods, 162
Minimal inhibitory concentration, definition, 12-13

Monensin, description, 66
Monitoring, definition, 137-138
Mycoplasmal disease control, by antibiotics, 53,55t

N

National Residue Program, duties, 137-138
Naturally occurring antibiotics in foods, lactic acid bacteria, 93-96
Negligible tolerance, definition, 129t
Neomycin, use in food animals, 19
Nisin, food preservative, 95-96
Nitrofurans, use, 3
Nonisotopic immunoassays, description, 150
<u>Nosema apis</u>, control by fumagillin, 45-46

O

Oral preparations of drugs
  dissolution rate, 15-16
  effectiveness, 16
Oxytetracycline
  federal regulations for use, 45
  label for use of Terramycin, 38t
  proper use, 39-43,44f,45
  stability in diets, 39-41t,42f,44f

P

Pad-plate procedure, 143
Penicillin
  efficacy, 16-17
  examples, 16
  use as feed additives, 4
Penzyme test, description, 148
Physicochemical methods for antibiotic residue determination
  chromatography, 155-163
  electrophoresis, 154-155
Plant growth promotion, by antibiotics, 56
Plant virus disease control, by antibiotics, 52-54
Polyether ionophores, description and usage, 66-67
Prolonged-release dosage form, advantages, 15

R

Radioimmunoassay, description and
 application, 150
Rationale for therapeutic use of
 antibiotics
 economic, 9
 problems arising from transfer of
 animals, 10
 treatment of whole group as an
 individual, 10
Regulatory aspects of antibiotics in
 agriculture
 approved antibiotics, 133t
 calculation of tolerance for a drug
 residue, 129,130t
 chronic toxicological
 testing, 123t,133
 concerns for residues of regulated
 antibiotics, 136
 consumption factors, 130t
 food additive amendment of 1958, 128
 Kefauver-Harris amendment of
 1962, 128
 minimum toxicological testing for an
 animal drug, 131,132t
 tolerance levels, 133t,134,136
 tolerances and toxicity tests, 129t
 violative residue rates, 130,131t
Residual antibiotics,
 effects, 91-92,93t
Residue avoidance feed test,
 description, 139
Routes of drug administration
 intravenous infusion, 14
 intramuscular and subcultaneous
 routes, 14-15
 oral preparations, 15-16
 prolonged-release dosage form, 15
 selection of dosage forms, 14
Rumen additives, 67-68

S

Salmonella resistance
 Chicago outbreak, 120-122
 English outbreak, 118
 Holmberg's findings, 122-123
 Illinois outbreak, 123
 Swann committee report, 118-119
 transferable resistance, 119
Second-generation cephalosporins,
 description, 17
Selection of antibiotics,
 factors, 11-13
Selective dry cow therapy for
 mastitis, criteria for
 success, 28,30

Streptomycin, use in food
 animals, 18-19
Subclinical mastitis, definition, 26
Subinhibitory concentration
 definition, 13
 effects, 13
Subtherapeutic levels, definition, 112
Sulfa drugs, use, 3
Sulfadimidine
 concentration ratios between tissue
 and plasma, 171,173t
 disposition, 171,175-176f,178f
 drug depletion time curves, 177,179f
 effect of metabolism, 180
 elimination half-lives vs. plasma
 protein binding data, 181
 experimental procedures for
 pharmacokinetic study, 169
 factors influencing persistance and
 pharmacokinetics, 181
 HPLC analysis, 169
 metabolic pathways, 169,170f
 molecular structures, 169,170f
 percentages in plasma of different
 species, 171,172t
 plasma concentration
 curves, 171,175f
 plasma disposition, 177,179f
 urinary recovery data, 171,174f
 urine concentration-time
 curves, 177,178f
Sulfamethazine
 tolerance level, 136
 use as feed additives, 4
Sulfathiazole, effectiveness against
 American foulbrood, 36,37f
Sulfonamide detection, by
 chromatographic
 methods, 155,156-157t,158
Sulfonamides, description, 20-21
Surveillance, definition, 138
Swab test
 description, 139
 types, 139-140
Swab test on premises,
 description, 139-140
Swab test on premises II,
 description, 140

T

Tests for antibiotic residues
 bioassays, 140
 chemical techniques and
 instrumentation, 141
 immunoassays, 140-141
 swab tests, 139-140
Tetracycline detection, by
 chromatographic methods, 158-159

INDEX

Tetracyclines
  description, 19-20
  use as feed additives, 3-4
Therapeutic use of antibiotics
  applications, 8-9
  rationale for use, 9
Third-generation cephalosporins,
  description, 17
Tissue penetration of a drug, 11
Tolerance for a drug residue,
  calculation, 129,130t
Trimethoprim, description, 20
Turbidimetric systems
  advantages and disadvantages, 146
  description, 145-146
Tylosin, use as feed additives, 4

V

Violative residue rates,
  values, 130,131t

W

Withdrawal period
  depletion curve for total residues
    of a drug, 134,135f
  methods to monitor residues, 136
Withdrawal time, definition, 117

Production by Joan C. Cook
Indexing by Deborah H. Steiner
Jacket design by Pamela Lewis

Elements typeset by Hot Type Ltd., Washington, DC
Printed and bound by Maple Press Co., York, PA

RECENT ACS BOOKS

Writing the Laboratory Notebook
By Howard M. Kanare
145 pages; clothbound ISBN 0-8412-0906-5

Plant Proteins: Applications, Biological Effects, and Chemistry
Edited by Robert L. Ory
ACS Symposium Series 312; 286 pp; ISBN 0-8412-0976-6

Phenomena in Mixed Surfactant Systems
Edited by John F. Scamehorn
ACS Symposium Series 311; 350 pp; ISBN 0-8412-0975-8

Chemistry and Function of Pectins
Edited by Marshall Fishman and Joseph Jen
ACS Symposium Series 310; 286 pp; ISBN 0-8412-0974-X

Fundamentals and Applications of Chemical Sensors
Edited by Dennis Schuetzle and Robert Hammerle
ACS Symposium Series 309; 398 pp; ISBN 0-8412-0973-1

Polymeric Reagents and Catalysts
Edited by Warren T. Ford
ACS Symposium Series 308; 296 pp; ISBN 0-8412-0972-3

Excited States and Reactive Intermediates:
Photochemistry, Photophysics, and Electrochemistry
Edited by A. B. P. Lever
ACS Symposium Series 307; 288 pp; ISBN 0-8412-0971-5

Artificial Intelligence Applications in Chemistry
Edited by Bruce A. Hohne and Thomas Pierce
ACS Symposium Series 306; 408 pp; ISBN 0-8412-0966-9

Organic Marine Geochemistry
Edited by Mary L. Sohn
ACS Symposium Series 305; 440 pp; ISBN 0-8412-0965-0

Historic Textile and Paper Materials: Conservation and Characterization
Edited by Howard L. Needles and S. Haig Zeronian
Advances in Chemistry Series 212; 464 pp; ISBN 0-8412-0900-6

Multicomponent Polymer Materials
Edited by D. R. Paul and L. H. Sperling
Advances in Chemistry Series 211; 354 pp; ISBN 0-8412-0899-9

For further information and a free catalog of ACS books, contact:
American Chemical Society, Sales Office
1155 16th Street N.W., Washington, DC 20036
Telephone 800-424-6747

LIBRARY OF DAVIDSON COLLEGE

ɔks on regular loan may be checked out for **two weeks.** Books
presented at the Circulation Desk in order to be renewed.

ged after date due.